ADVANCES IN EYE RESEARCH

ADVANCES IN EYE RESEARCH

VOLUME 1

ADVANCES IN EYE RESEARCH

Additional books in this series can be found on Nova's website under the Series tab.

Additional E-books in this series can be found on Nova's website under the E-books tab.

ADVANCES IN EYE RESEARCH

ADVANCES IN EYE RESEARCH

VOLUME 1

WILLIAM L. THOMSEN
EDITOR

Nova Science Publishers, Inc.
New York

For permission to use material from this book please contact us:
Telephone 631-231-7269; Fax 631-231-8175
Web Site: http://www.novapublishers.com

Additional color graphics may be available in the e-book version of this book.

Library of Congress Cataloging-in-Publication Data

ISBN: 2162-3295

ISBN 978-1-61324-169-1

Published by Nova Science Publishers, Inc. † New York

Contents

Preface

This new series presents original leading edge results in the field of eye research. The focus in this compilation is on the anatomy of the cornea as well as the causes, symptoms and treatments for uveitis. Topics discussed include conjunctival-limbal autografts; gene therapy for corneal diseases; uveitis in juvenile idiopathic arthritis; retinal vasculitis in rheumatic disease; Vogt-Koyanagi-Harada disease and the clinical and immunopathological highlights of non-infectious uveitis.

Chapter I - Limbal stem cell transplantation is the definitive treatment for the limbal stem cell deficiency. The type of surgery depends on the laterality and severity of the condition. In the case of unilateral total LSCD, conjunctivel limbal autograft (CLAU) and cultivated limbal epithelial transplantation (CLET) are the main surgical options. The long-term anatomical results and visual outcomes of CLAU are excellent. Subsequent penetrating or lamellar keratoplasty may be needed for visual rehabilitation. The most important risk factors for graft failure are severe dry eye, chronic inflammation and associated adnexal abnormalities. The most important complications are related to transplanted limbal lenticules.

Chapter II - The World Health Organization estimates that 45 million people worldwide are suffering from blindness. Corneal and other ocular surface diseases are the 3rd leading cause of global blindness. Conventional treatments are effective but associated with significant side effects that can undermine their clinical utility. Gene therapy is an emerging innovative technology for eye disease treatment and prevention. The successful restoration of vision in a few human patients outlines its enormous potential in treating eye disorders. Gene therapy may potentially treat genetic and acquired corneal blindness due to scarring, graft rejection, angiogenesis, dystrophies, keratitis, Sjogren syndrome, and ocular surface disorders. Gene therapy entails the use of novel vectors to transfer therapeutic genes into corneal cells to modulate the expression of a particular protein, growth factor, or cytokine that in turn will modify corneal disease. Two major determinants for the success of gene therapy are the use of an appropriate vector and gene delivery technique. Numerous viral vectors such as adenovirus, adeno-associated virus (AAV), lentivirus, and retrovirus, as well as nonviral vectors such as lipid, gold nanopariticle, dendrimer and different catatropic polymers have been tested for ocular diseases. Each of these vectors has its own advantages and limitations. Recently, next generation AAV vectors were developed by creating a point mutation that increased transgene delivery into the retina 15-30 fold at 10 fold less doses. Our ongoing studies with these next generation mutant AAV vectors and gold nanopariticle nonviral vectors suggest that these delivery systems are 10-25 fold more efficient than conventional viral and nonviral vectors for delivering genes in the cornea in animal experimental models.

Chapter III - In view of the extensive use of radioactive isotopes in medical fields such as nuclear diagnostics (computerized tomography), nuclear medicine, radiation dosimetry and radiation biophysics, the knowledge on X- and gamma ray interactions with different types of materials has become the subject of researches for nuclear engineers, radiologists and radiation physicists for different purposes i.e. shielding, dosimetry, X-ray imaging and radiotherapy. The photon mass attenuation and mass energy absorption coefficients, energy dependence, effective atomic number, effective electron density and buildup factor are the basic quantities required in determining the penetration of X- and gamma photons through the material. While the extensive studies based on radiation interaction in biological materials are available, there are almost no studies for soft contact lenses from the point of X- and gamma ray interactions. At this point, the present study aimed at the investigation of X and/or gamma radiation interaction with different types of soft contact lenses in terms of the parameters viz. mass attenuation and energy absorption coefficients, effective atomic number, effective electron density and energy dependence in the wide energy range of 1 keV-20 MeV as well as the energy absorption and exposure buildup factors from 0.015 to 15 MeV up to 40 mfp penetration depth. The influences of photon energy, chemical composition and penetration depth on these parameters were studied.

Chapter IV - Uveitis, an important manifestation of various autoimmune diseases and of some infectious disease, is a multifactorial disease. Children constitute 5-10% of the patients with uveitis seen at tertiary referral centers. The most common cause of anterior uveitis is idiopathic juvenile arthritis (JIA). The diagnosis and management of chronic pediatric uveitis can be particularly challenging, with an estimated 25-33% of childhood uveitis cases resulting in severe, life-long visual disability due to ocular complications such as cataract, band keratopathy, glaucoma and cystoid macular edema. Although infectious uveitis, once properly identified, may be successfully treated by addressing the inciting organism with specific therapy, the immune-mediated chronic forms of uveitis often provide more complex challenges in management. In addition uveitis associated with autoimmune diseases may be refractory unless the underlying systemic disease is adequately treated.

The aim of this chapter is to review uveitis in JIA and discuss possible treatment strategies.

Chapter V - Retinal vascular inflammation, a potentially blinding condition (herein: retinal vasculitis - RV) is commonly associated with a heterogeneous group of diseases characterized by systemic inflammatory cell infiltration and/or necrosis of blood vessel walls. RV may arise as a primary or secondary disorder (rheumatoid arthritis, Wegener's granulomatosis, polyarteritis nodosa) or it can be secondary to an underlying collagen disease, systemic refection or malignancy. Depending on the type of RV, it can be potentially blinding; in the short or long term. Early diagnosis is the key to successful treatment and better prognosis. However, early diagnosis can be difficult, because these conditions usually present with non-specific visual symptoms for a long period before diagnostic manifestations occur.

RV can be detected clinically (often accompanied by uveitis, scleritis, macular edema) or revealed on fluorescein fundus angiography, even if minimal clinical and ophthalmologic signs of retinal vessel inflammation are present. Therefore the retina should be examined in warranted patients with rheumatic disease, since retinal vasculitis may be asymptomatic at the beginning (peripheral retinal disease). RV can also represent one of the possible extra-articular manifestations of the rheumatic disease. Rheumatologists should be familiar with the ocular manifestations of these disorders, since they may not only be sight threatening, but more importantly, could be the presenting – or even the very first manifestations of active, potentially lethal systemic disease in a patient with non specific rheumatologic presentation.

Chapter VI - Uveitis is a generic term used to describe intraocular inflammation occurring anywhere within the eye. It arises from a diverse group of diseases and is commonly classified based on its location within the eye as anterior, intermediate, posterior, or panuveitis. This review focuses on noninfectious or autoimmune uveitis and its associated immunopathology. Intraocular inflammation can be acute or chronic. Acute inflammation is marked by infiltration of neutrophils and macrophages while chronic inflammation is marked by infiltration with lymphocytes and macrophages. From an immunopathologic perspective intraocular inflammation can be further studied by the dominating inflammatory cells and their subsets, their inflammatory products including cytokines and immunoglobulins, and the ocular resident cells whose own cell surface markers and adhesion molecules are altered by inflammation. By describing the clinical features of noninfectious uveitis and correlating it with its underlying immunopathology, it will hopefully lead to further clarification of the immunopathogenesis.

Chapter VII - The term panuveitis is reserved for diseases that involve all segments of the uveal tract, including the retina and vitreous body. It is usually associated with severe sight-threatening inflammatory response. The common causes of panuveitis in our population are tuberculosis, syphilis, Vogt-Koyanagi-Harada disease, sympathetic ophthalmia, Behçet's disease and sarcoidosis. Vogt-Koyanagi-Harada disease (VKH) is a multisystem autoimmune disorder affecting pigmented tissues such as the eye, auditory, integumentary and central nervous systems. Patients are typically females between 20 to 50 years old with no previous history of penetrating ocular trauma. Despite the increasing reports published about the clinical features of VKHdisease in various ethnic populations, the etiology of VKH disease is still not completely known. Clinical, laboratorial, experimental data corroborate to the autoimmune nature of VKH disease in a genetically susceptible individual. A stepwise approach is essential while evaluating these patients to be able to identify and treat the disease timely and adequately. Ancillary tests can be appropriately applied once the clinical diagnosis is made. Treatment is based on initial high-dose oral corticosteroids with a low tapering during a minimum period of 6 months. Systemic immunomodulatory agents such as cyclosporine may be used in refractory or corticosteroid non-tolerant patients. Visual prognosis is usually good under a prompt diagnosis and adequate treatment. The aim of this paper is to review the latest research results on VKH disease in order to help to understand better this potentially blinding disease and to improve treatment.

Chapter VIII - The eye is an essential organ for survival and is highly vulnerable to the destructive potential of immunogenic inflammation. Immune privilege of the eye has coped with the countermanding threats to vision of ocular infections and ocular immunity and inflammation. Among the primary features that account for its existence is the anterior chamber-associated immune deviation with a prolonged acceptance of solid tissue and tumor allografts in the anterior chamber and the induction of systemic tolerance to eye-derived antigens. Therefore, immune-mediated inflammation in the eye does not develop at the same pace as in other sites of the body. Uveitis is the most common autoimmune manifestation that affects the eye and may be an important cause of blindness among young individuals. The autoimmune nature of several uveitis is supported by experimental data from animal models, the presence of *in vitro* T lymphocytes responses to one or more retinal auto-antigens, the association of specific HLA molecules and the responsiveness to immunosuppressive drugs. Acute anterior uveitis is the main ocular manifestation of spondyloarthropathies in which uveitis can be the first manifestation of the disease. Precise patterns of uveitis are frequently associated with systemic diseases. Thus, the close collaboration between ophthalmologists and rheumatologists avoids unnecessary diagnostic tests and is essential for the correct assessment and treatment of these patients. Acute anterior uveitis usually has a good prognosis compared with other forms of uveitis. However, it is a cause of disability when flares are frequent. Small prospective studies conducted with sulphasalazine have demonstrated a reduction in the number of flares. Other patterns of uveitis have a worse prognosis, and systemic corticosteroids and/or immunosuppressive drugs are usually required.

The aim of this paper is to review the main rheumatological conditions associated with uveitis and discuss possible treatment strategies for these conditions.

In: Advances in Eye Research. Volume 1 ISBN 978-1-61324-169-1
Editor: William L. Thomsen, pp. 1-46

Chapter I

Conjunctival-Limbal Autograft (CLAU)

Medi Eslani,[1] Alireza Baradaran-Rafii,[2] Alireza Djalilian[3]

[1]School of Medicine, Tehran University of Medical Sciences, Tehran Iran
[2]Ophthalmic Research Center, Shahid Beheshti University of Medical Sciences, Tehran, Iran
[3]Department of Ophthalmology and Visual Sciences, University of Illinois at Chicago, Chicago, IL, USA

Abstract

Limbal stem cell transplantation is the definitive treatment for the limbal stem cell deficiency. The type of surgery depends on the laterality and severity of the condition. In the case of unilateral total LSCD, conjunctivel limbal autograft (CLAU) and cultivated limbal epithelial transplantation (CLET) are the main surgical options. The long-term anatomical results and visual outcomes of CLAU are excellent. Subsequent penetrating or lamellar keratoplasty may be needed for visual rehabilitation. The most important risk factors for graft failure are severe dry eye, chronic inflammation and associated adnexal abnormalities. The most important complications are related to transplanted limbal lenticules.

Limbal Stem Cells

The ocular surface consists of a continuous epithelial layer and its overlaying tear film. It can be divided into three distinct zones of the cornea, the limbus and the conjunctiva. The general organization of the limbal and conjunctival epithelia is the same as that of the corneal epithelium. However, there are some important differences; for example the conjunctival stroma is vascular whereas the corneal stroma is avascular [1] and mucin-secreting goblet cells can be found in the conjunctival epithelium unlike the cornea and the limbus. [2]

The limbus is a thin transitional zone which divides the peripheral cornea from the conjunctiva. [2] There is a high ratio of basal to superficial epithelial cells at the limbus. The basement membrane becomes discontinuous and undulating. It forms the "palisades of Vogt," which are thought to provide a protective environment for maintenance of stem cells which is necessary for the regeneration of the corneal epithelium. [3] Molecular mechanisms for regulating limbal epithelial stem cells remain unclear despite cumulative evidence indicating that their function is influenced by their surrounding microenvironment; "the limbal stem cell niche". [4-9] These poorly differentiated, slow cycling cells have great capacity for colonogenic expansion and error-free division with a long life-span. These cells, which act as a barrier against corneal conjunctivalization, are dependent on factors such as limbal stroma (niche), tear production and conjunctival vasculature. [5, 8, 10]

There is strong evidence supporting the concept that stem cells at the limbus serve to replenish corneal epithelium. [3, 11-13] In healed eccentric corneal epithelial defects in heavily pigmented eyes, pigmented epithelial migration lines (cells) that migrate from the limbal region towards the central cornea are observed.(3] Proper corneal wound healing is impaired when the limbal epithelium is partially or completely removed. [13-19] When a significant portion of the limbus is lost, the corneal surface is covered with conjunctival epithelium by a process referred to as conjunctivalization. [20] Restoration of the limbal epithelium by transplantation can restore the normal corneal epithelium. [21, 22] A critical mass of limbal epithelial cells is necessary to compete with the conjunctiva for re-epithelialization of a denuded corneal surface.

The generally accepted model of corneal re-epithelialization involves limbal stem cells (LSCs) undergoing asymmetric cell division to give rise to two daughter cells, one that starts on the path of differentiation as a "transient amplifying cell" and one that remains undifferentiated in order to maintain the stem cell pool. These transient amplifying cells migrate centripetally to populate the basal layer of the corneal epithelium and then they give rise to the postmitotic epithelial cells that differentiate into the terminally differentiated cells of the epithelial surface. [23]

Corneal epithelial cells continually shed from the corneal surface and have an average lifespan of 4 to 6 days. [3, 20] They are constantly generated by cell division at the basal epithelial layer and by centripetal movement of cells from the peripheral limbus to the central cornea. [24] The corneal epithelium also has a remarkable capacity to heal itself. Superficial epithelial cells migrate into corneal defects and small surface abrasions usually heal rapidly without complication. [20, 23] This migration is followed by an increase in basal cell mitotic activity away from the wound site, as well as an increase in proliferation of limbal epithelial basal cells. The cells that have migrated into the wound attach themselves to the basement membrane and proliferate to fill the epithelial defect. [3, 23, 25]

Stem Cell Deficiency

Ocular surface failure can be categorized into two major types. Corneal conjunctivalization (limbal failure) as a manifestation of LSCD constitutes one major type of ocular surface failure leading to corneal blindness (Figure 1). It is the process of corneal coverage by in-growing conjunctival epithelium containing goblet cells, which was originally thought to provide the restoration of a normal corneal epithelium via the process of conjunctival transdifferentiation. [26, 27] However, the epithelium regenerated from corneal cells and epithelium regenerated from conjunctival cells have major biochemical and functional differences. [18, 28] One other major type of ocular surface failure is caused by squamous metaplasia which is mainly caused by severe dry eye, where corneal as well as conjunctival epithelia turn into a stratified, non-secretory, keratinized epithelium. Such ocular surface failure is evident by the cellular hyperproliferation, stratification and keratinization of the ocular surface. [9, 29]

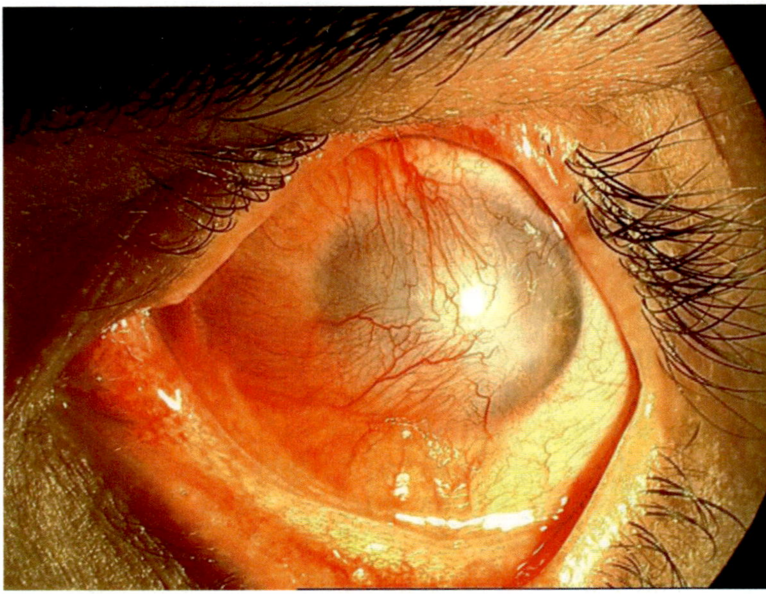

Figure 1. Type I ocular surface failure with severe stem cell deficiency.

It is important for the clinician to understand the proportional contribution of LSCD and conjunctival disease in selecting the surgical options for a patient's rehabilitation. Staging is determined by status of both the limbal stem cells and conjunctiva. [31] Partial LSCD can be classified as stage I; while total LSCD can be classified as stage II. If conjunctiva is normal, the patient is staged as "a," and if the conjunctiva is abnormal, the patient is staged as "b." Therefore, total LSCD with normal conjunctiva would be in stage II a, whereas total LSCD with abnormal conjunctiva will be staged as II b. Iatrogenic LSCD, [35] contact lens induced keratopathy and conjunctival intraepithelial neoplasia are examples of conditions that fit the classification of stage Ia. Patients exhibiting stage I a disease can progress to II a with further loss of limbal stem cells. The conditions mentioned above, in addition to aniridia, can also progress to stage II a. [31, 36-38] Patients with mild to moderate conjunctival disease can develop subsequent partial LSCD (Stage Ib), such as conjunctival inflammatory disorders that have not reached the severe stage; for example, mild Stevens–Johnson syndrome, ocular cicatricial pemphigoid; and chemical injuries. Conjunctival inflammation may lead to conjunctival scarring, aqueous tear deficiency and the eventual loss of partial limbal function. The most severe form of ocular surface disease with the poorest prognosis (stage II b) includes severe Stevens–Johnson syndrome, ocular cicatricial pemphigoid and chemical injuries. In these cases, total LSCD is complicated by conjunctival scarring, decreased aqueous and tear production and potential for keratinization of the ocular surface. [31, 39]

Table 1. Causes of Limbal Stem Cell Deficiency

Primary limbal stem cell deficiency (Hereditary)		
Aniridia		
Epidermal dysplasia	ectrodactyly-ectodermal dysplasia-clefting syndrome	
Congenital erythrokeratodermia	Keratitis-ichthyosis-deafness syndrome	
multiple endocrine deficiencies		
Idiopathic		
Secondary limbal stem cell deficiency (Acquired)		
Chemical, thermal, or mechanical injury		
Stevens-Johnson syndrome/TEN	toxic epidermal necrolysis	
Ocular cicatricial pemphigoid		
Iatrogenic	medication toxicity	mitomycin C or 5-FU
	surgical trauma	Multiple surgeries or cryotherapies to limbus
Radiation	Ultraviolet or ionizing	
Pterygia/pseudopterygia		
Chronic limbitis	vernal, atopic, phlyctenular	
Chronic bullous Keratopathy	Superior limbic keratoconjunctivitis	
Collagen vascular diseases		
Contact lens-induced keratopathy		
Severe microbial infection extending to limbus		
Peripheral ulcerative keratitis (Mooren's ulcer)		
Limbal neoplasms		

Clinical Manifestations

Limbal stem cell deficiency is associated with conjunctivalization of the cornea. The clinical symptoms of limbal deficiency may include decreased vision, photophobia, tearing, blepharospasm and recurrent episodes of pain (epithelial breakdown), as well as a history of chronic inflammation with redness. Biomicroscopic examination at the slit-lamp may show the corneal epithelium having a dull, opaque and irregular reflex with variable thickness. The loss of the limbal palisades of Vogt is also another feature, [33, 40] but it should be borne in mind that the palisade architecture of the limbus is not uniform through the circumference of the limbus. The presence of distinct palisade architecture in some segments and a complete absence in others is consistent with normal limbal function. However, the loss of the palisades of Vogt after an injury, in an area known to have the palisade architecture before the injury, is very indicative of stem cell loss. In some cases, a mosaic pattern, representing an admixture of the two cell types, can be seen on the corneal surface when the corneal and conjunctival epithelial phenotypes are not well demarcated. [41] It can be complicated with recurrent and persistent epithelial defects, superficial corneal vascularization, irregular epithelium, scarring, calcification, ulceration, melting and perforation of the cornea. Besides conjunctivalization, limbal deficient corneas also carry other pathologic features, such as destruction of the basement membrane, emergence of superficial neovascularization, chronic stromal inflammation and scarring. Because the conjunctival epithelium is more permeable than corneal epithelium, [16] the conjunctivalized corneal surfaces are frequently stained abnormally by fluorescein (delayed fluorescein staining). [33, 34, 42]

Diagnosis

"Conjunctivalization" is the most reliable diagnostic sign of the limbal deficiency, because vascularization and inflammation can also be seen in other corneal diseases. [33, 40] This phenomenon can be detected bio-microscopically and also by delayed fluorescein staining. The use of impression cytology provides confirmation, [26, 43-45] which can detect goblet cells containing conjunctival epithelium on the corneal surface. [26] Impression cytology is a useful non-invasive technique, in which the first or the two outermost layers of the ocular surface epithelium are removed and studied to determine the state of the epithelial surface. It is the gold standard for confirmation of the conjunctivalization of the cornea. Finding goblet cells on the surface of the cornea is considered the definitive diagnosis for corneal conjunctivalization and LSCD. [26] It can also be combined with immunocytochemistry evaluation. [46, 47] Even if impression cytology is used, in conditions such as severe chemical burn, cicatricial ocular pemphygoid or Stevens–Johnson syndrome the conjunctival goblet cells, which are detectable by PAS staining, are not always detected in patients with clinically suspected LSCD. [9, 26, 48] Although, it has been suggested that in vivo confocal microscopy can be helpful in the diagnosis of LSCD. [9, 48] A future challenge rests on delineating a biomarker that is expressed not by cellular differentiation present on the suprabasal layers (such as goblet cells or keratinization), but by stemness inherently present at the basal stem cell level.

Management of Stem Cell Deficiency

Management of LSCD depends on the extent of involvement (partial or total), laterality (uni or bilateral), severity of ocular surface inflammation, presence of symblepharon, tear status, ocular surface keratinization and systemic factors such as age and the general health of the patient. [32, 49, 50] The only definitive treatment for LSCD is Limbal stem cell transplantation. The main objective is to continue to supply a new corneal epithelium for a prolonged, if not indefinite, period of time so that patients can be relieved from annoying photophobia and regain useful visual acuity. A specific and widely accepted modified nomenclature for different techniques of limbal stem cell transplantation has been proposed by Holland and Schwartz. [5, 51]

Partial Limbal Stem Cell Deficiency

The management of partial LSCD aims at helping the remaining healthy LSC population to expand. In unilateral cases, limbal stem cell transplantation (LSCT) is not usually required if the patient can be kept under close observation. [41] The patient's vision is usually good when the visual axis is covered with epithelial cells with corneal phenotype, but only conservative treatment is suggested if the patient is otherwise asymptomatic. [32, 33, 41] Topical lubrication may be helpful to prevent corneal epithelial erosions. Healing of the cornea and conjunctiva should be allowed to occur by their respective phenotype of cells. Patients with partial stem cell deficiency with irritation, decreased vision (usually when the visual axis is covered with conjunctival epithelial cell phenotype) or persistent epithelial defects may require surgical intervention.

Sequential Sector Conjunctival Epitheliectomy; SSCE

Dua and coworkers [42] initially reported the technique of mechanical debridement of conjunctival epithelium from the corneal surface under topical anesthesia. [33] The key to the success of this technique is close monitoring of the patient after the debridement to ensure that healing of the denuded corneal surface occurs from the remaining corneal epithelium and not from the conjunctival epithelium. The principle of preventing the conjunctival epithelium from reaching and crossing the limbus applies equally in this situation. Dua, [41] later reported a high rate of success in a series of patients in whom this principle was applied in the management and prevention of partial stem cell deficiency. This principle of close monitoring of the healing of the conjunctival epithelium and preventing it from crossing the limbus is also the key to success of auto- and allo-limbal transplants, particularly where sectors or segments of limbal tissue have been transplanted. Tseng et al [33] reported successful management of patients with sector LSCD by mechanical debridement of conjunctiva- like epithelium from the corneal surface, but combined the procedure with amniotic membrane transplantation.

Amniotic Membrane Transplantation

In cases with partial limbal deficiency, AMT alone may suffice to prevent and postpone limbal transplantation. It is shown in several studies that in eyes with partial LSCD, AM promotes the expansion of remaining limbal epithelial stem cells. [52-55] In this surgery following the removal of conjunctivalized pannus from the corneal surface AM is transplanted and fixed either by sutures or fibrin glue. [56]

Total Limbal Stem Cell Deficiency

The main determinant of the type of LSC graft used is whether the LSCD is unilateral or bilateral. Unilateral cases with total LSCD may benefit from either a conjunctival-limbal autograft (CLAU) or transplantation of cultured limbal stem cells from the healthyfellow. In bilateral conditions with total LSCD, an allograft limbal transplant utilizing donor tissue from a cadaver (keratolimbal allograft; KLAL) or a living relative (living-related conjunctival-limbal allograft; lr-CLAL) are the main options. If an HLA-matched donor is available, lr-CLAL may be preferable because in theory, there will be less need for systemic immunosuppression. However, systemic immunosuppression is necessary after either procedure. [57] CLET is an alternative. If the LSCD is bilateral, but there are some remaining unaffected regions, it may be possible to culture autologous cells from healthy areas of the limbus. Another recently introduced option is the use of ex vivo cultured oral mucosal epithelial cells (cultivated oral mucosal epithelial transplantation; COMET). (Flowchart 1)

AMT has been shown to be complementary to any type of limbal transplantation. It can be used in conjunction with or preceding limbal transplantation for most situations in which the latter is used. Because only substrate and no live cells are transplanted, allograft rejection does not occur with AMT. The basement membrane facilitates migration of epithelial cells, [52] it reinforces adhesion of basal epithelium, [53] promotes cellular differentiation [54] and prevents cellular apoptosis. Collectively, these actions are conducive to rapid epithelialization. The amniotic membrane matrix suppresses the TGF- signaling system, DNA synthesis and the subsequent myofibroblast differentiation. [55] These actions decrease scarring. Facilitation of epithelialization, decreased inflammation and decreased scarring collectively provide a milieu that promotes success of limbal transplantation if both of the procedures are performed concurrently and encouraging clinical results have been obtained with this approach. [56, 58, 59] To eliminate the concern of removing excessive limbal epithelium, amniotic membrane can also be used in the healthy donor eye in conjunction with CLAU and lr-CLAL. [60] AMT has been advocated as the first-stage procedure to be followed by limbal epithelial transplantation at a later stage, because after AMT perilimbal conjunctival tissues become less inflamed and retain healthy conjunctival surface quality. This approach has the advantage of providing a stromal microenvironment favorable to survival of limbal tissues. [56]

Conjunctival Limbal Autograft (CLAU)

In the case of unilateral total LSCD, a conjunctival-limbal autograft, which first reported by Kenyon and Tseng [61] and experimentally confirmed by Tsai et al. may be considered [22] If partial LSCD is not managed fully by conservative measures, then LSCT with CLAU may also be used. Ipsilateral translocation to an area of partial LSCD (ipsilateral CLAU) has been shown to have a good outcome in a small series of patients with limited LSCD. [32, 62, 63] The therapeutic role of CLAU has also been demonstrated for ocular burns, [64-75] in the surgical management of pterygium, [63, 76-82] after excision of limbal masses, [83] after repeated surgeries [84] and in contact lens– induced keratopathy [74]. [85]

Living-related Conjunctival Limbal Allograft Transplant (lr-CLAL)

When total LSCD is bilateral, corneal surface reconstruction relies on transplantation of allogeneic limbal epithelial stem cells. To do so, one option is to transplant lr-CLAL from living-related donors. The surgical procedure of lr-CLAL is identical to CLAU. Nevertheless, unless the donor and the recipient are perfectly matched, the success of lr-CLAL depends on systemic immunosuppression and allograft rejection is still the main threat. [86]

Keratolimbal Allograft Transplant (KLAL)

The other option is to perform keratolimbal allograft (KLAL) from cadaveric donors. This surgical technique was first reported by Tsai and Tseng [87] and has since been reported by others. [6, 88] KLAL may restore limbal stem cells in patients with bilateral LSCD or in patients with unilateral LSCD, who do not wish to expose the healthy eye to any surgical procedure or have any comprised condition in seemingly healthy eye. It is mandatory to administer systemic immunosuppression as in lr-CLAL. [6]

Cultivated Limbal Epithelial Transplantation (CLET)

Another procedure is ex vivo expansion of autologous [89-91] or allogeneic [92, 93] limbal stem cells, which was first demonstrated by Pellegrini et al. [94] This new surgical procedure is effective in achieving a limbal epithelial phenotype on the corneal surface. [6, 91] The theoretical advantage of ex vivo expansion over CLAU and lr-CLAL is that only a small limbal biopsy is needed, thus minimizing the risk to the donor eye. The theoretical advantage over KLAL and lr-CLAL is that the allograft rejection might be reduced as only epithelial cells are transplanted and antigen-presenting Langerhan's cells are eliminated during ex vivo expansion. This surgical procedure can be used in cases with unilateral or bilateral total stem cell deficiency. In the unilateral cases, the source is a healthy fellow eye and in bilateral cases, the source can be living-related or cadaveric eyes. [6, 92, 93]

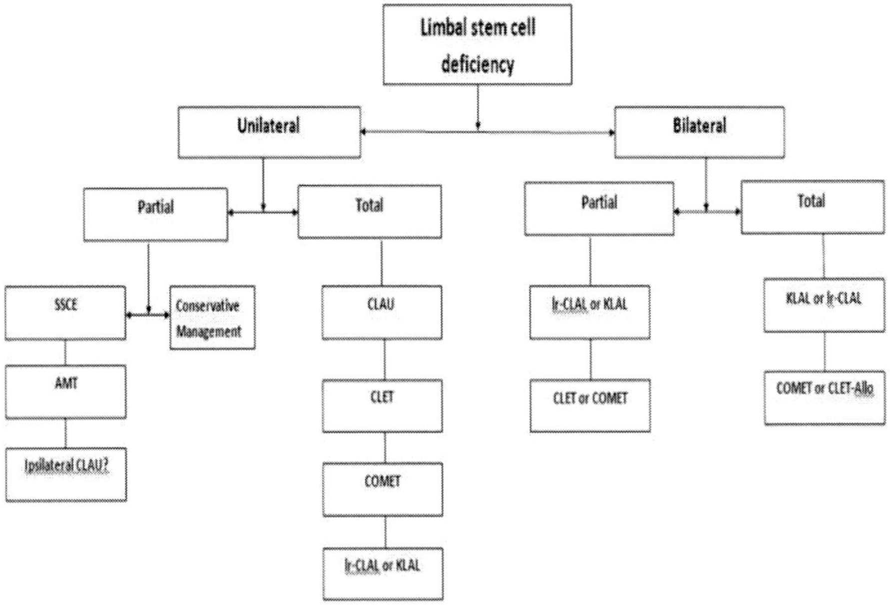

Flowchart 1. Management of the stem cell deficiency.

Ocular Surface Optimization and Adnexal Reconstruction

Most of the patients with total LSCD have also associated lid structural abnormalities and tear film problems. Stem cells have to be permanently covered by a continuous layer of tear film. It is well-known that exposure, dry eye and inflammation are very important risk factors for the survival of the stem cell grafts. [10, 49] Aqueous and mucin tear deficiency, subepithelial fibrosis, symblepharon, ankyloblepharon, foreshortening of the conjunctival fornices and in most severe cases, keratinization of the entire surface will compound ocular surface disorders. [31]

Ocular surface inflammation has a well-known detrimental effect on the survival of limbal stem cells. Conjunctival disease in combination with limbal stem cell disease will result in the most severe form of ocular surface disease. Co-existing stromal inflammation is an unhealthy microenvironment for the survival of the transplanted limbal stem cells. [68] In the acute and subacute phases of severe chemical burns, inflammation should be minimized to allow the cornea to be completely conjunctivalized and vascularized with minimal symblepharon formation without corneal perforation. Inflammation should also be minimized after surgery. Systemic steroids may be helpful. Running conjunctival sutures or fibrin glue is preferred. To have a tight apposition between transplanted stem cells and the cornea, the corneal and scleral sutures should be interrupted, long, tight, inert and buried. To minimize inflammation even more, 10-0 nylon sutures are preferred.

Fornix reconstruction is very important before stem cell transplantation. In the case of small symblepharon bands, it can be done at the time of transplantation surgery. The conjunctival mantle of donor limbal lenticule should be spread and sutured to the recipient ocular surface. Large symblepharon bands and diffuse fornix shortage will lead to a dry and inflamed ocular surface with high amounts of discharge. Fornix reconstruction can be performed using autologous conjunctiva from the fellow eye, amniotic membrane or mucosal grafts with or without mitomycin-C (MMC). [95, 96] Using mucosal grafts is sometimes necessary due to extensive symblepharon formation. Also in corneas impending to perforation, mucosal grafts may provide tectonic support leading to final vascularization of the cornea.

It is advisable to perform fornix reconstruction a few months before transplantation. Lid structural abnormalities should also be corrected as much as possible prior to surgery. Small lid notches sometimes cause chronic exposure. This may lead to progressive conjunctivalization, thinning/ perforation, chronic stem cell attrition and final failure. Care should be taken to avoid heavy cauterization of scleral bed to prevent scleral thinning/melting, staphyloma formation, glaucoma occurrence and finally losing the eye in cases with severe chemical burns and ischemia.

What is important and should be considered before performing stem cell transplantation include preliminary measures such as trichiatic lashes removal, using bandage contact lenses, tear film normalization by emollients, transient or permanent punctal occlusion and tarsorrhaphy. [10, 50] These measures can provide symptomatic improvement in mild cases, especially in the presence of adequate transient amplifying cells in the center of the cornea. Undue surgery or administration of eye drops containing preservatives should be avoided as much as possible in these cases. [10] If extensive symblepharon lysis is required, application of mitomycin C 0.02% using non-dripping sponges for 3 to 5 minutes within the subconjunctival recesses followed by copious irrigation prior to fornix reconstruction is useful for preventing recurrent symblepharon.

Glaucoma management in patients with LSCD is difficult. Preoperatively, the intraocular pressure should be controlled. The use of glaucoma drainage devices preoperatively has been suggested. [56] In the event of postoperative raised intra ocular pressure, a shunt may be needed since conjunctival scarring precludes performing trabeculectomy. As a last option, cyclodestructive procedures may be carried out in an eye with poor visual potential.

Preoperative Evaluation

Complete eye examinations including visual acuity measurement, biomicroscopic examination, intraocular pressure measurement and funduscopy should be performed. B-scan ultrasonography is needed for eyes with severe haziness of ocular media to rule out gross posterior segment pathologies. Where the fundus is not visible or the visual potential can not be clinically ascertained, electrophysiologic tests (visual evoked potential and electroretinography) should be performed and adequacy of tear film should be evaluated using tear meniscus height and Schirmer's test. Eye examination should also be thoroughly performed in all potential fellow eyes. If there is any noticeable ocular disease such as glaucoma (probability of future trabeculectomy) or history of long-term contact lens use (probability of future limbal failure), they should be excluded. Integrity of corneal and conjunctival epithelium should be evaluated by vital dyes including fluorescein, rose Bengal and lissamine green stains. [9, 32, 33]

Stem cell deficiency should be confirmed using impression cytology. It is a useful non-invasive technique, in which the first or the two outermost layers of the ocular surface epithelium are removed and studied to determine the state of the conjunctival surface. This is the gold standard for confirmation of the conjunctivalization of the cornea. Finding goblet cells on the surface of the cornea is considered the definitive diagnosis for corneal conjunctivalization and LSCD. [26]

In patients with severe unilateral chemical injury, it is not uncommon for the fellow eye to sustain subclinical injury. [65] Although casual examination reveals a normal corneal and ocular surface, careful slit lamp biomicroscopic evaluation of the inferior limbus may reveal a subtle alteration or loss of the palisades of Vogt. Absence of these pigmented ridges is a sign of damage to the limbus and stem cells. [13] Due to the protective Bell's phenomenon, the inferior limbus is more prone to such damage. Evidence of such damage should be considered a relative contraindication for limbal stem cell autografting. Preoperative impression cytology of the donor epithelium is useful in situations in which there is a suspicion regarding integrity of the stem cells.

Surgical Procedure

Donor Eye

Two 60-degrees arcs of limbal lenticule, each spanning 6–7 mm length are harvested from 12 and 6 o'clock positions, starting with lamellar dissection in the cornea 1 mm anterior and extending 2 mm posterior to the limbus, leaving behind as much of the Tenon capsule as possible. Lamellar dissection can also be started on the conjunctiva and carry forward towards the limbus about 1-1.5 onto the cornea in a very superficial manner. A 5 mm conjunctival mantle is simultaneously harvested to help fornix reconstruction in the injured eye. The amount of the conjunctiva can be increased if the recipient eye also requires symblepharon correction. At the end, conjunctiva is dissected, advanced and fixed exactly to the limbal area without any corneal coverage with 10-0 nylon sutures. Care should be taken to avoid damage to the limbus by buttonholing or dessication of the donor tissue during excision. Although the donor sites heal quickly, sutures should be placed in the lateral margin of each site to enhance patient comfort and confidence. The defect can also be covered by AMT.

Recipient Eye

Surgery is done under general or peribulbar anesthesia. After a 360-degree conjunctival peritomy, shaving of sclera is done. Hemostasis is achieved with mild wet-field cautery or dilute adrenaline (1:10,000). Subconjuntival scar tissues are removed as thoroughly as possible, which invariably results in the recession of the conjunctival edge to 3–5 mm from the limbus. In the case of extensive subconjunctival scar formation, mitomycin-C 0.02% is applied to the adjacent conjunctival fornix for 3 minutes and then is thoroughly irrigated with balanced salt solution. Corneal pannus is removed totally using a crescent knife with special caution not to perforate cornea. Using BP blade # 11, a partial thickness (30% depth) rectangular corneoscleral bed including 1 mm of cornea and 2 mm of adjacent sclera may be prepared, however this may not be necessary if the donor grafts are sufficiently thin. The exposed ocular surface is thoroughly covered by cryopreserved amniotic membrane, sticky stroma side down. Amniotic membrane is fixed to the ocular surface with fibrin glue or 2 running 10-0 nylon sutures at the limbus and 3.0 mm away. It is also sometimes sutured to the peripheral conjunctiva and episclera. Donor lenticules with nearly the same dimensions should be transferred to the prepared bed and separately sutured to the recipient eye at the corresponding anatomic sites by interrupted 10-0 nylon sutures to the limbus and 8-0 vicryl sutures to the sclera, aligning limbal areas together. The CLAU grafts can also be directly glued to the prepared bed with fibrin glue. For prevention of symblepharon formation and deepening of fornices, donor and recipient conjunctivae are sutured. The surgical site is usually covered with an overlay amniotic membrane or a high DK bandage contact lens. At the end of surgery, upper and lower punctal occlusion and lateral tarsorrhaphy should be performed to protect grafts from the mechanical trauma of blinking as well as from evaporative moisture loss in the early postoperative period in most of the cases.

Most reports [63, 65, 76, 97] describe the removal of donor limbus with an underlying bed of carrier corneal stroma of varying thickness. Others [66, 77] describe the removal of limbal tissue by the progressive undermining of the conjunctival flap onto the corneal surface until the vascular arcades are reached. The dissected tissue is then excised using Vannas scissors, thereby avoiding corneal stromal dissection. Anatomical and functional outcomes of the latter technique have been reported as very good in the recipient eyes with no report of the occurrence of conjunctivalization of the donor sites. [85]

Postoperative Management

The basic principles of postoperative management for any LSCT procedure are control of inflammation, prophylaxis against infection and assurance of adequate ocular surface lubrication. Normally, two waves of progressive epithelial healing appear in front of the transplanted lenticules 1 to 2 days after surgery. They usually reach together after 7-14 days. (Figures1-A and 1-B) Using amniotic membrane as a graft provides a better means of evaluating progressive epithelialization over the ocular surface by donor limbal epithelial cells.

After surgery, oral prednisone 1mg/kg/day is started and tapered off over 6-8 weeks as the inflammation decreases. Topical antibiotic and steroid drops (preferably preservative-free) should be started after surgery 4-6 times a day. The former is discontinued when corneal epithelialization is complete, while the latter is tapered off according to ocular surface inflammation during 6 to 8 weeks. Topical steroids can be continued longer on a low maintenance dose. Excessive treatment in the early postoperative period is better to be avoided as to avert the retardation of epithelialization. [98] Autologous serum drops are sometimes used and should be tapered off in 2-3 months. Instead of serum drops, topical preservative-free artificial tears are sometimes administered. Lubrication of the ocular surface should then be continued using topical preservative-free artificial tears and lubricating gels or ointments. If there is elevated intraocular pressure, topical or systemic antiglaucoma medications should be used.

As for partial stem cell deficiency, it is important to monitor the patient closely during the healing process and to ensure that conjunctival epithelium does not encroach onto the corneal surface even in total stem cell deficiency. Re-epithelization of the cornea should be allowed to occur from cells derived from the transplanted limbal tissue only. [33, 99] Sequential epitheliectomy can be used to remove invading conjunctival epithelium. Monthly follow-ups are needed to monitor recurrence of conjunctivalization and ocular surface breakdown. High DK bandage soft contact lenses may be used in the early post operative period for 6-8 weeks. In long-term follow-up, if the tear film is somehow compromised or there is mild exposure, using high DK lenses may help patient to have a constant spread of tear film over the corneal surface. They can also be used to alleviate discomfort from the long-standing PEE and

PEKs. [5] Small lateral tarsorrhaphy (cosmetically acceptable) can also help improve cases with persistent epitheliopathy.

Outcomes and Results

The healing of corneal epithelial defects and appearance of a smooth transparent epithelial surface with regression of opacity, vascularization and thinning are considered as the components of clinical success. Failure is the appearance of persistent epithelial defect (nonhealing epithelial defect longer than two weeks) with progressive corneal vascularization and thinning.

Clinical assessment of the ocular surface health on a diseased cornea by corneal epithelial transparency and degree of vascularization is subjective and prone to misinterpretation. [100, 101] Detecting conjunctivalization over a diseased cornea is difficult. The corneal epithelium is irregular and the stroma is opaque and vascularized; therefore, the optical contrast is not enough to easily determine the wave of slowly progressive conjunctivalization. However, after subsequent lamellar or penetrating keratoplasty, tracking the superficial wave of conjunctivalization and vascularization is more convenient.

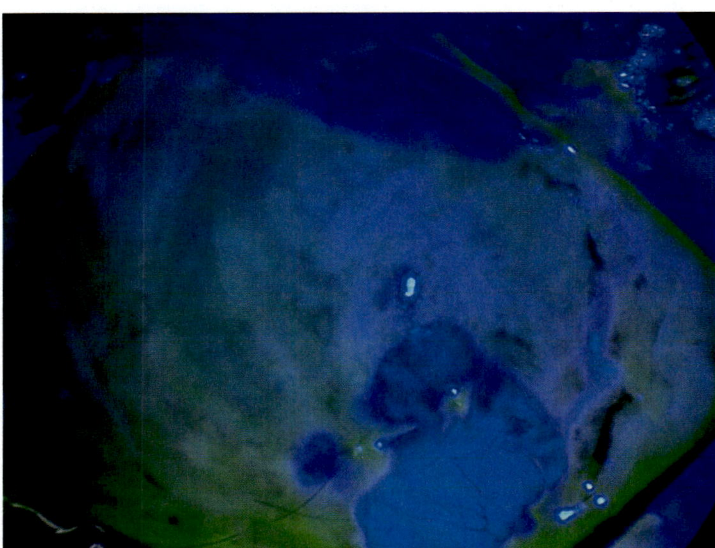

A

Figure 2. (Continued).

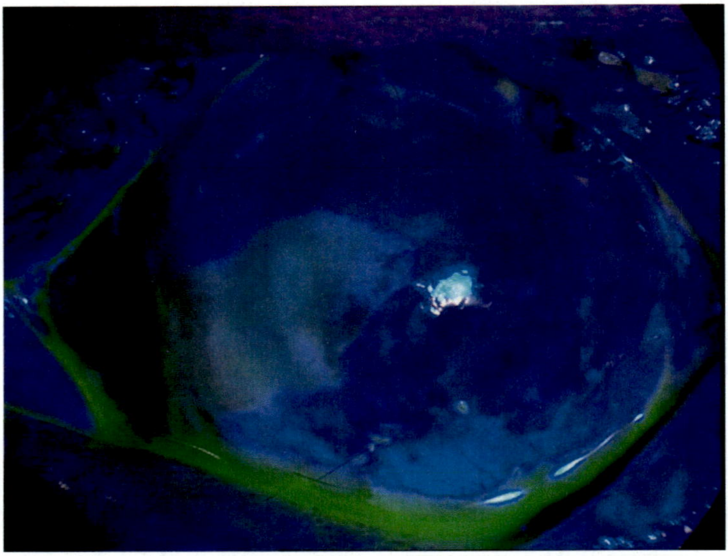
B

Figure 2. A: Two waves of progressive epithelial healing is shown in front of transplanted limbal lenticules. B: Note to progressive epithelial waves 7 days after surgery.

A number of studies (which in most cases are series) have shown overwhelming (greater than 80%) successful visual outcomes with regression of neovascularization and improvement of corneal transparency after CLAU. (Figures 2-A, 2-B, 2-C) [60, 61, 66, 69, 72, 101-104] More than 20 years of follow-up experience with CLAU cases demonstrates excellent long-term improvement in the eyes that received LSC grafts and no serious complications in the LSC donor eyes. [23]

In general, there have been very few reports of complication and success rates of CLAU for unilateral LSCD have been excellent. [32] Corneal reepithelialization usually occurs between days 7 and 28 and regression of stromal neovascularization is evident soon thereafter. [23, 61, 66, 102] In Kenyon and Tseng's original report, [61] patients who were followed for at least 6 months had stable ocular surfaces without epithelial defects and 17 of 21 had improved visual acuity. Rao and colleagues [66] reported success in 15 of 16 patients and similar success rates have been reported in other small case series as well. [60, 69, 72, 101-104]

In spite of successful corneal epithealialization and regression of vascularization, limiting factors such as refractive errors, corneal scars, cataract formation, amblyopia and corneal epithelial disintegrities usually decrease their BSCVA. [23, 32]

Graft Survival

Almost all studies on CLAU report the results on recipient eyes with short-term and intermediate follow-up periods. [60, 61, 66, 69, 72, 73, 101-104] The question regarding the maintenance of the function of transplanted limbus over the long term is presently unanswered and what has been disturbing is that some studies have reported attrition in function in some recipient eyes. [65, 74, 105] These studies provide suggestive evidence that transplanted tissue can show a temporal decrease or even loss of function. This information should be borne in mind when offering patients the option of CLAU and during prognostication.

It is well known that stem cell transplantation has limited survival rates, especially of the allogenic or cadaveric types. [101, 106] Stem cells die gradually due to acute or chronic immunologic rejections or other offending mechanisms, such as unstable tear film, exposure problems (incomplete blinking, reduced blinking rate, lagophthalmos and lid margin notching), mechanical injurys (trichiasis, distichiasis, keratinization of the lid margin, cicatricial entropion or ectropion and symblepharon), shallow fornices, conjunctival irregularity, probable improper stem cell niche and other unknown factors. [5, 32, 107, 108] These can lead to chronic cell attrition which is the main cause of failure after CLAU. In the case of conjunctival encroachment onto the cornea, entrapment of limbal cells may prevent corneal epithelialization. This may finally lead to failure and should be corrected promptly.

CLAU in Pterygium

The CLAU graft is almost always taken from the non-affected superior limbus of the ipsilateral eye when used to treat pterygium. [78, 109] In preparing the recipient area, only limited superficial keratectomy of the head of the pterygium plus resection of the involved conjunctival and Tenon's tissue is required. The conjunctival autograft is then secured with either sutures or fibrin adhesive. For pterygium treatment, outcomes of CLAU as well as standard conjunctival autograft [78] have been excellent and in fact, superior to the use of amniotic membrane grafting alone; recurrence rates of pterygium after CLAU have ranged from 0% to 7%. [110-114] In a randomized prospective trial, CLAU with amniotic membrane grafting was demonstrated to be superior to intraoperative mitomycin-C treatment with amniotic membrane grafting. [113] Multiple studies suggest that for management of primary as well as recurrent pterygia, both conjunctival autograft and CLAU have the same results. They are both less costly and complication-prone than amniotic membrane grafting, with or without mitomycin-C. CLAU, although interesting, does not represent an improvement over the use of simple conjunctival autograft transplantation for pterygium and hence at this point seems to be a somewhat costly "overtreatment." [23]

Prognostic Factors

Patient selection, counseling of recipients and potential donors, close postoperative monitoring and multiple interventions (both medical and surgical) are keys to the success of limbal transplantation. The success of limbal transplantation may be adversely affected by concomitant lid pathology, dry eye, ocular surface keratinization, chronic inflammation, uncorrected lid and lid margin abnormalities, timing of surgery, subclinical donor cell disease and uncontrolled systemic disorders. [64, 65] Hence, the management of LSCD also involves the management of associated adnexal conditions, dry eye and systemic diseases; [6, 106, 115] among all, severe dry eye and chronic inflammation are the most important risk factors. [101]

In the acute phase of chemical burns, fluorescein staining involving the limbus does not ascertain that limbal stem cells have been completely destroyed at the basal level. Persistent inflammation has been recognized as a major threat leading to LSCD in humans. [26, 68] Without effective measures to suppress inflammation (steroids, AMT and etc), even healthy limbal stem cells will surely decline; let alone if they are already compromised by the aforementioned injury maladies. Patients with chronic inflammatory causes of LSCD have worse outcomes with ocular surface reconstruction and LSCT than do patients with acute, non-inflammatory causes of LSCD. [100, 116, 117] For chronic conditions, the ongoing injuries to the LSC niche from chronic inflammation, sicca or other immune-mediated complications are more likely to result in recurrent LSCD even following otherwise successful transplantation. Generally, inflammation should be aggressively controlled before and after surgery.

What has been identified as the most important prognostic factor on the surgical outcome and survival of limbal transplantations is the severity of dry eye. [101] Generally, LSCT should be avoided in patients with moderate to severe forms of dry eye. In the mild forms of dry eyes, ocular surface lubrication should be maximized before stem cell transplantation.

It is critically important to diagnose patients with LSCD properly, because they are poor candidates for conventional corneal transplantation. In eyes even with quiescent LSCD (e.g., many years after a chemical burn), performance of lamellar or penetrating keratoplasty only replaces the host's corneal epithelium temporarily without addressing the lack of LSCs. In such cases, the additional surgical stress (e.g., severing corneal nerves in the process of trephination) can perpetuate neurotrophic components and precipitate epithelial defects, stromal neovascularization and ultimate graft failure.

Appropriate timing of the surgery is very important. In chemical burns, severe inflammation and ischemia in the acute stage is a threat to the success of transplanted CLAU. Amniotic membrane transplantation has been suggested as a temporary patch to suppress inflammation, facilitate epithelial wound healing and prevent scarring in acute burns [118] and Stevens–Johnson syndrome/toxic epidermal necrolysis. [119] It is generally suggested not to perform CLAU if the limbus is avascular and to consider measures such as tenonplasty to facilitate vascularization of the limbal bed before performing CLAU in eyes with severe limbal ischemia. As a fact, visual outcomes are poorer in eyes with earlier surgery even after complete re-epithelialization. It is not yet clear whether this is because of recurrent conjunctivalization or stromal factors. [22] Based on clinical experience available at this time, it is clear that CLAU is optimally performed in eyes that are not inflamed and have well vascularized limbal beds.

Some surgeons now believe that preoperative impression cytology of the donor cornea is prudent, even in eyes that may otherwise appear clinically normal, to rule out subclinical donor cell dysfunction. The presence of goblet cells on the cornea suggests decreased stem cell function. [120] For the same purpose, eyes that have even a suspicion of damage, based on history or clinical examination are best not be used as donors. [65] Therefore, unilateral partial limbal compromise after chemical burns should never be treated with

CLAU from a seemingly healthy looking limbus from the same eye. It is important to harvest tissue from the other eye in such cases.

Complications

Traditionally, two 60-degrees limbal lenticules have been used to repopulate the ocular surface. Though excision up to eight clock hours has been recommended, the optimum amount of limbal tissue that may be harvested from the donor eye has not been determined; thus, it is wise not to remove large amounts of the limbus. [32, 121] Excision and transplantation of more than six clock hours is best avoided for fear of precipitating LSCD in the donor. Amniotic membrane as a niche may decrease the minimum necessary size of limbal lenticules. It is yet unknown how these donor eyes will respond to an epithelial injury in the future, thus a conservative removal may be prudent. Experimental evidence shows the development of LSCD in a rabbit model. [13, 14] Despite this concern, reports regarding subsequent stem cell deficiency in a healthy donor eye, are very rare and it seems that in the case of a good patient selection, it is a safe and uneventful procedure. [107] More studies with long term results are awaited as failure due to stem cell attrition ascribed to inflammation and subclinical donor cell disease has been reported. [9, 64, 85] Because of poor tear film quality and disturbances in its distribution over the ocular surface, conjunctival and forniceal shortage and the lid structural abnormalities; these patients have an unstable ocular surface with probable future chronic cell attrition. Therefore, they need enough permanent stem cell reserves for a long-term stable ocular surface. Using two limbal lenticules combined with AMT may be necessary to have a long-term stable ocular surface.

Intraoperative complications of the recipient eye include damage to the muscle during symblepharon release, bleeding during superficial keratectomy and corneal perforation. Epithelial complications include chronic and recurrent PEE, PEK and PEDs. These epithelial disintegrities are more common after subsequent PKP or LKP. It should be noted that the cause of PED should be carefully identified. PED could be due to stem cell deficiency, ocular surface exposure, dry eye and toxic medications. In each condition, the cause should be corrected. The predisposing factors of epithelial breakdown include persistent or severe inflammation, [86, 122] lid abnormality, [99] contact lens induced keratopathy, [64] trichiasis [92] and following applanation tonometry. [32, 123] Healing may be hastened by frequent instillation of preservative-free topical lubricants, autologous serum and hyaluronic acid. [63, 99] Botulinum induced ptosis has successfully been used for the management of persistent epithelial defects. [56] Conjunctival encroachment onto the cornea, leads to entrapment of limbal cells which can prevent corneal epithelialization. This would finally lead to PED, sectoral conjuctivalization and vascularization and finally failure. It should be corrected promptly.

In most situations, putting limbal blocks at 6 and 12 o'clock positions is important in maintaining a constant coverage by upper and lower lids with a good spreading of tear film. Chronic exposure will lead to thinning, progressive vascularization and final failure of donor lenticules. Limbal blocks should be adequately trimmed and thinned. Putting up thick limbal lenticules would be a barrier for proliferated epithelial cells to pass the step and cover the ocular surface. It also may result in improper distribution of the tear film with subsequent dellen formation. [32] Applying amniotic membrane as a graft may be helpful for filling up the step between thick or poorly trimmed limbal blocks and the ocular surface.

Limbal alignment is important for preventing exposure and cutting lenticules during trephination in probable future keratoplasty. Choosing a proper size trephine with a good centeration is important. Cutting limbal lenticules will produce an iatrogenic partial stem cell deficiency and final failure (Figures 3-A and 3-B). Small lenticules should also be avoided. This may lead to PED, sectoral conjunctivalization, thinning and perforation after CLAU or subsequent PKP. (Figures 4) Proper suturing and timely suture removal are necessary to prevent dislodging of the donor tissue by the shearing action of the lids and to avoid injury to the growing epithelial edge. Friction due to lid movement and loose sutures may dislodge lenticules (Figure 5).

Glaucoma management in patients with LSCD is difficult. Preoperatively the intraocular pressure should be controlled. The use of Seton drainage devices preoperatively has been suggested. [56] In the event of postoperative raised intra ocular pressure, a shunt may be needed since conjunctival scarring precludes performing trabeculectomy. As a last resort, cyclodestructive procedures may be carried out in an eye with poor visual potential.

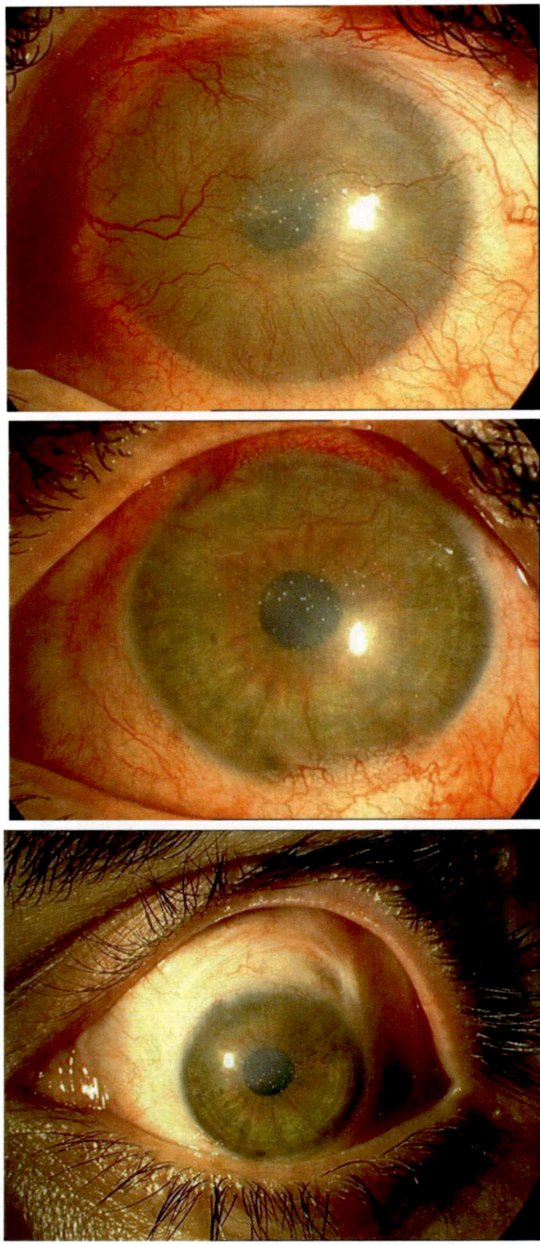

A

B

C

Figure 3. A: A patient with unilateral severe vascularization and opacification of the cornea due to chemical burn. B: 6 months after CLAU. Note decreasing vascularization and opacification of cornea with increase transparency. C: 2 years after CLAU.

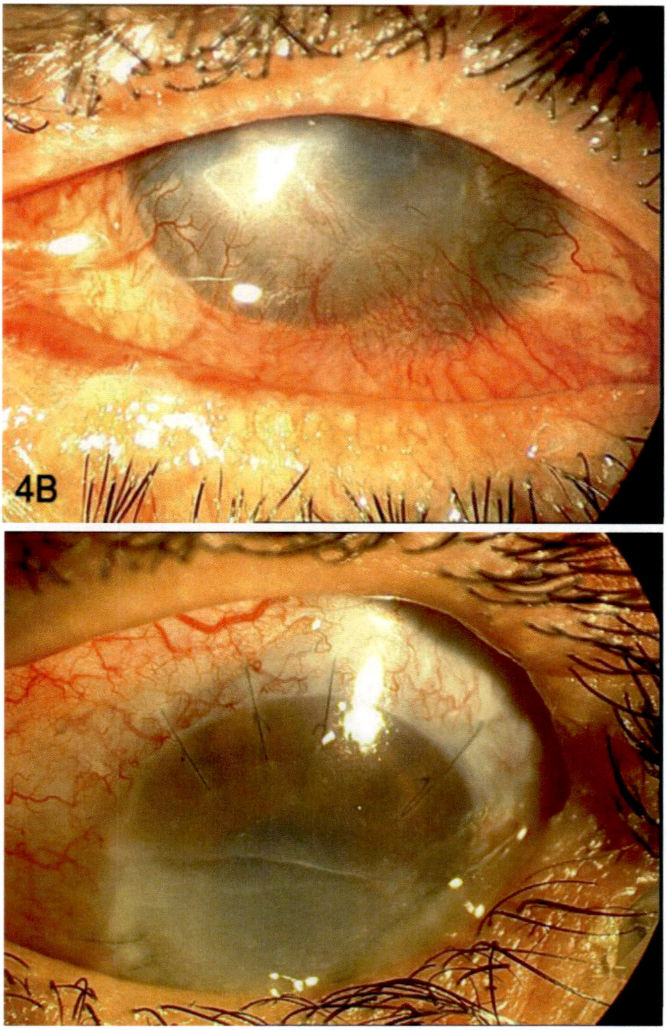

A

B

Figure 4. A: Localized vascularization and opacification of the cornea due to iatrogenic partial stem cell deficiency after unplanned trephination of limbal lenticule. B: persistent epithelial defect after PKP due to unplanned trephination of inferior limbal lenticules.

In some cases, progressive horizontal conjunctivalization and vascularization are evident. This may be due to insufficient transplanted stem cells. (Figure 6) Although infective keratitis is quite rare following limbal stem cell transplantation, if it occurs aggressive antimicrobial therapy is necessary.

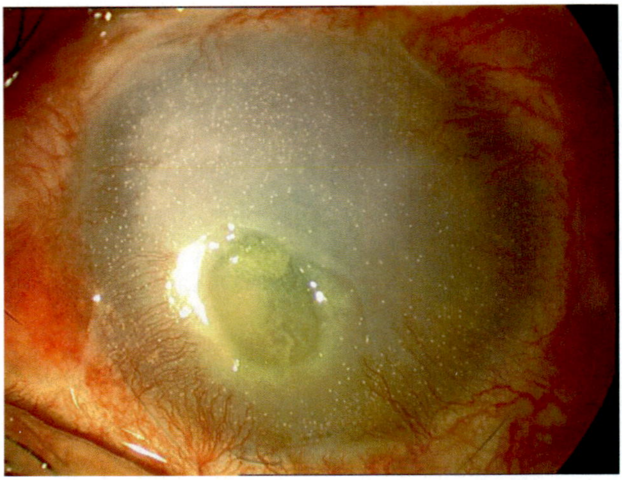

Figure 5. Persistent epithelial defect due to inferior small transplanted lenticule.

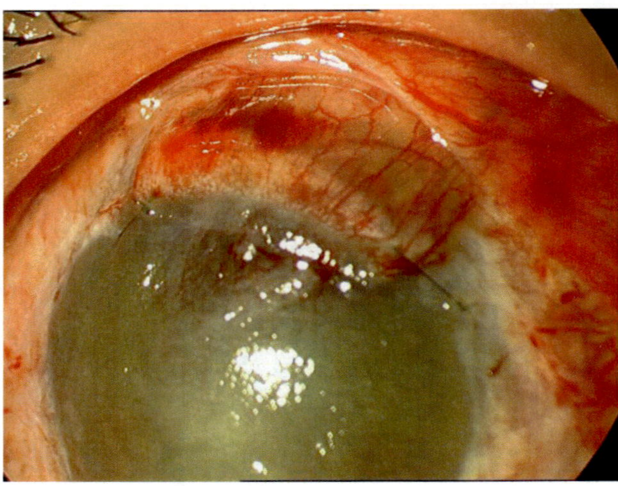

Figure 6. Dislodging of the superior limbal lenticule due to premature suture removal and shearing action of the upper lid.

Donor Eyes Complications

Several complications have been noted in donor eyes including localized haze, [102] pseudopterygium, [74, 82] filamentary keratitis, [66] microperforation during surgery, [65] abnormal epithelium, [124] progressive conjunctivalization and corneal depression. [64] Although it is generally believed that the donor eyes with such limbal removal recover well without complication, scattered reports show that some donor eyes may become complicated by pseudopterygium or partial LSCD, especially in eyes with subclinical LSCD. One alternative to preclude such a potential complication is to transplant amniotic membrane as a graft to cover the defect after removal of CLAU in the donor eye and over the corneal surface before CLAU in the recipient eye, so that the remaining and transplanted limbal epithelial stem cells can be expanded in the donor and recipient eye, respectively. [60]

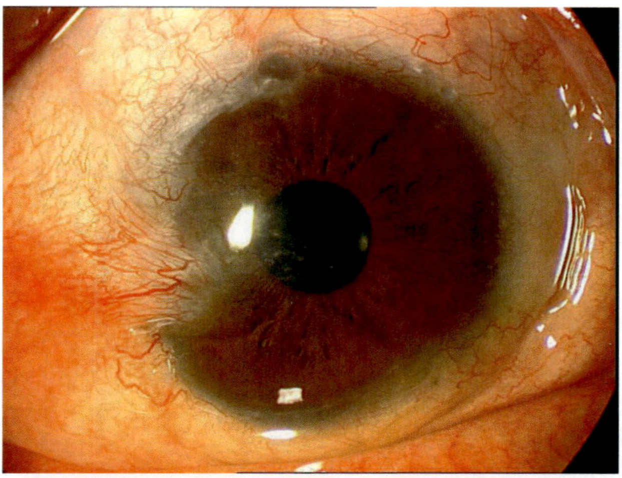

A

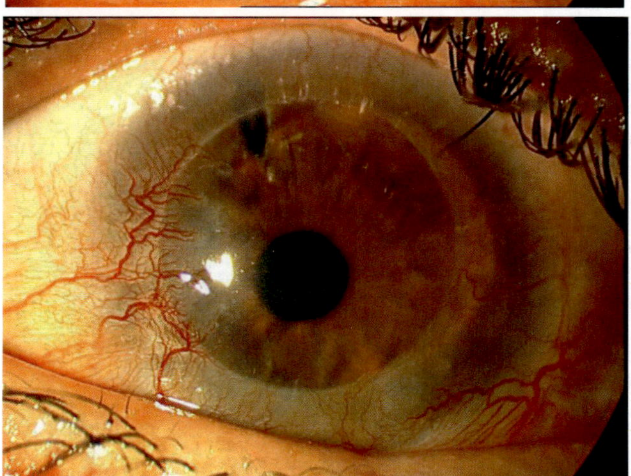

B

Figure 7. A: Progressive horizontal vascularization and conjunctivalization of the cornea. B: progressive conjunctivalization in the subsequent PKP after CLAU.

Subsequent Corneal Transplantation

Accurate diagnosis and grading of the severity is crucial for planning an effective surgical strategy for LSCD. Although correct diagnosis of LSCD leads to successful visual rehabilitation, less appreciated is that casual diagnosis of LSCD without cytologic confirmation can be detrimental by subjecting the patient to unnecessary transplantation of limbal stem cells.

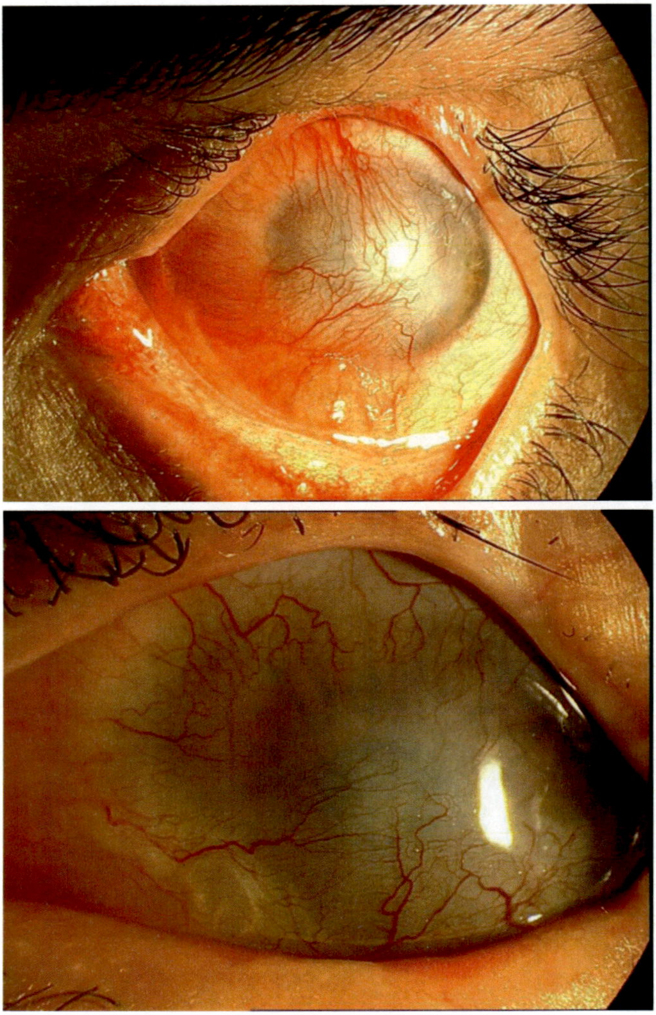

A

B

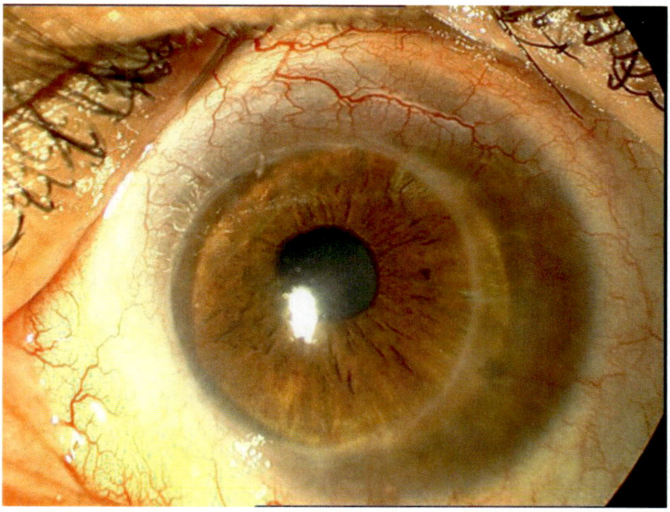

C

Figure 8. A: A case of total unilateral stem cell deficiency due to severe chemical burn. B: Note to decreased vascularization and opacification of the cornea 6 months after CLAU. C: Subsequent PKP was performed to clear visual axis.

Many superficially scarred corneas will regain remarkable clarity with visual improvement following LSC grafting alone. For those eyes with deeper stromal opacity or corneal edema, it is best to add corneal transplantation 3 or 4 months later when the eye is not as inflamed. In this manner vision is restored with a clear cornea. To further minimize corneal graft rejection, another solution is to perform deep lamellar keratoplasty rather than penetrating keratoplasty especially when there is no corneal endothelial dysfunction. (Figures 7-A, 7-B and 7-C) [49, 106, 107, 125]

There are some challenges during corneal transplantation in these cases. Heavy recipient corneal stromal vascularization causes intraoperative intracameral hemorrhage and decreases the surgeon's view. Applying phenylephrine 5% or diluted epinephrine drops leads to pupillary dilation and anterior displacement of crystalline lens during suturing. In patients with high positive vitreous pressure anterior displacement of crystalline lens may occur. Recipient cornea is sometimes very thin. Non-homogenous stromal structure and low corneoscleral rigidity may cause anterior segment collapse during surgery.

There are some surgical points regarding PKP after CLAU. Intraoperative cauterization is better to be avoided to prevent wound shrinkage and wound leakage. In this procedure, it is preferable not to manipulate the eye. Trying to have a deeper anterior chamber during surgery may lead to more endothelial cell loss, recurrent hemorrhage and wound problems. It should be tried to form the anterior chamber in the early days after surgery using anti-inflammatory drugs and cycloplegics to facilitate intracameral hemorrhage absorption. Performing multiple surgical peripheral iridectomies is important to prevent peripheral anterior synechiae formation, decrease the chance for air-bubble or clot-induced acute angle closure glaucoma and reduce the chance for peripheral anterior synechiae formation and probable future chronic angle closure glaucoma. Sutures should be separate with tight and long bites. Due to severe thinning of recipient cornea in some areas, full-thickness suturing is sometimes unavoidable. Irregularity in the recipient-donor junction may lead to wound leakage; this may necessitate additional suturing. Care should be taken not to include iris stroma into the suture bites. Toxic suture reaction and cheese-wiring are common complications. Due to concomitant ocular surface disorders, small diameter corneal buttons are preferred. At least, 0.5mm graft disparity should be considered in all cases to ensure adequate anterior chamber depth. In the case of a heavy vascularized recipient cornea and compromised ocular surface, PKP or LKP may be considered as high risk. Therefore, in some cases using systemic immunosupression may be helpful for increasing donor cornea survival.

For mild immunosuppression in some patients with highly vascularized beds or recurrent corneal graft rejections, systemic immunosuppression using cyclosporine A, mycophenolate mofetil, tacrolimus etc. is needed. Care should be taken to avoid systemic adverse events and complications such as nephrotoxicity, hepatotoxicity, hypertension, neurotoxicity and etc. The dose of immunosuppressives should be adjusted and monitored in collaboration with an immunosuppression expert.

Using a good quality donor cornea with a healthy epithelial layer is important. Corneal epithelial defect in the presence of a compromised ocular surface or a borderline stem cell population predisposes the donor cornea to PED, corneal thinning and perforation. Having a good healthy epithelium over donor cornea gives the cornea opportunity to be slowly vascularized with minimal thinning. Epithelial healing after PKP or LKP may be more complicated. In the presence of a borderline stem cell reserve or mild exposure in an eye without significant epithelial problems after CLAU, PED may occur after PKP due to neurotrophic component and surface irregularities. Long standing and recurrent PEE and PEK after CLAU, especially after PKP or LKP are common findings in these eyes. [5] This may cause annoying foreign body sensation, redness and tearing. They are due to infrequent and incomplete blinking, lids structural abnormalities, tear film disturbances and an uneven ocular surface. They will finally lead to poor tear film distribution and epithelial disintegrity. [32, 50]

A good coverage of epithelium over the donor corneal graft in the acute stage after corneal transplantation is not a good indicator for a sufficient reserve of stem cells. It mostly depends on the donor cornea epithelial layer. In the case of a borderline or insufficient stem cell reserve, epithelial problems including punctate epithelial erosions and transient epithelial defects would develop. It may ultimately lead to PED, corneal thinning and perforation.

Surgical Alternatives

Cultivated Limbal Epithelial Transplantation (CLET) and Cultivated Oral Mucosal Epithelial Transplantation (COMET)

In the event of unilateral total LSCD, transplantation of cultivated autologous limbal stem cells from the healthy fellow eye is another alternative. Cultivation of a small part of the limbus may provide epithelial progenitor cells which may survive for awhile. There have been a number of reports on ex-vivo expanded autologous LSCT with different follow-up periods (Figures 8-A, 8-B, 8-C and 8-D). [107, 126-128] In almost all studies, the authors conclude that this method is a successful procedure to treat unilateral corneal stem cell deficiency. Whether results with CLET are comparable to the time-tested outcomes of CLAU, needs more investigations.

Ex vivo expansion has the advantage of requiring only a small piece of donor tissue (especially when it is from the other unaffected eye or a living relative), reducing potential risks of donor site complications. However, this requires specialized expertise and a licensed laboratory, can take up to 2 weeks to generate a sheet of desired dimensions and is more expensive. Therefore, Limbal transplant of the donor tissue or “in vivo expansion” still remains a viable and cost-effective option. [129]

The exact proportion of stem cells presented in ex-vivo cultured limbal epithelial cell sheets is unclear and needs to be determined. The behavior of limbal epithelial stem cells post-transplantation needs to be elucidated. It has been proposed that the success of this treatment relies on the re-integration of exogenous cultured limbal stem cells into the ocular surface and thus these cells function to continuously replenish the corneal epithelium. Stem cells in CLAU are located on their natural niche, while cultivated presumed progenitor cells are located over the AM which is considered a potential niche.

Most recently, oral mucosal epithelial cells have been cultured on amniotic membrane, used to treat severe ocular surface disorders. [128] These oral explants do not have LSCs, but they seem to be a source of LSC equivalents that are able to generate cornea-like epithelium under the proper culture conditions. The main advantage of oral mucosal epithelial cell grafts that are cultured ex vivo is that patients with bilateral LSCD can be treated with grafts derived from their own autologous oral mucosal cells.

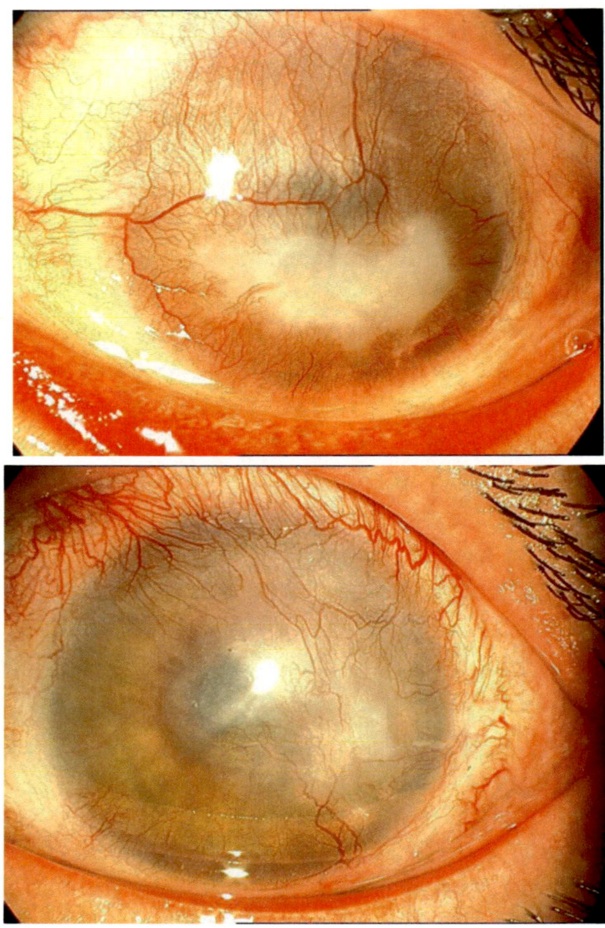

A

B

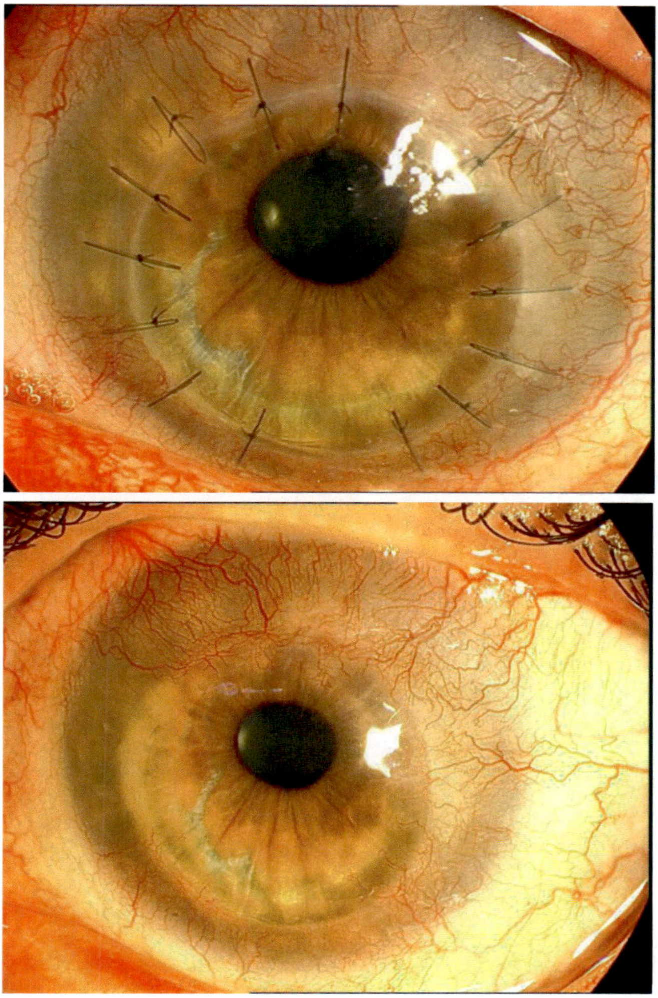

C

D

Figure 9. A: A case of unilateral total stem cell deficiency. B: 4 months after successful CLET. C: 2 months after subsequent PKP. D: Mild progressive conjunctivalization and vascularization of the transplanted cornea 1.5 years after surgery.

Due to fully-established long-term results of CLAU, [130] higher amounts of transplanted stem cells, more physiologic niche, lower risk of gradual cell attrition, uncertainties regarding the optimized method of cultivation, unknown nature of the cultivated growing cells, indefinite long-term clinical outcomes and the cost of the cultivation, CLAU remains the treatment of choice for most of the cases with unilateral LSCD.

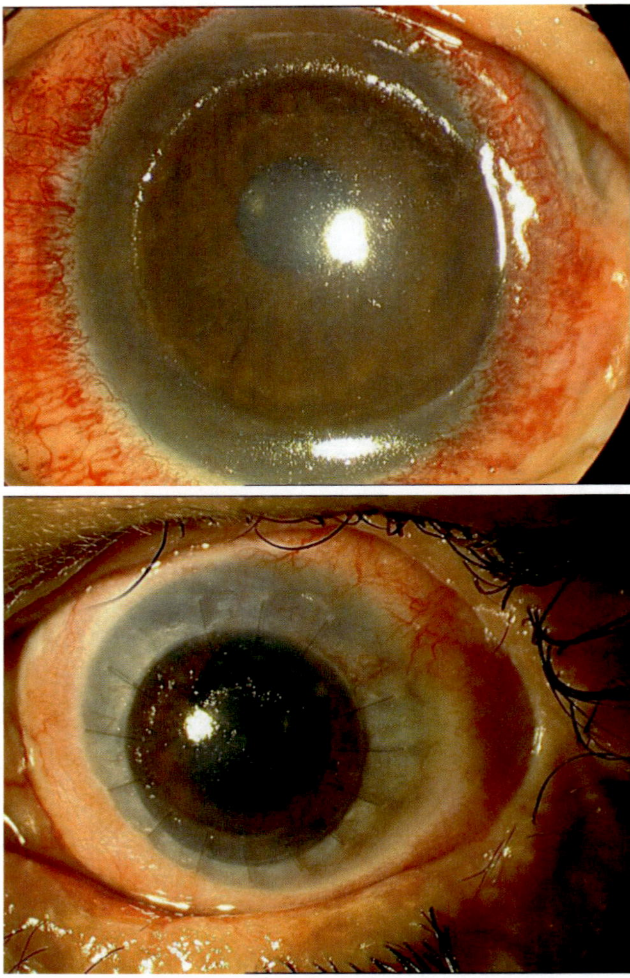

A

B

Figure 10. A: Successful KLAL in a case with bilateral severe chemical burn. B: Subsequent PKP in another case after successful KLAL with dense opacification of the cornea.

There are some surgical points regarding PKP after CLAU. Intraoperative cauterization is better to be avoided to prevent wound shrinkage and wound leakage. In this procedure, it is preferable not to manipulate the eye. Trying to have a deeper anterior chamber during surgery may lead to more endothelial cell loss, recurrent hemorrhage and wound problems. It should be tried to form the anterior chamber in the early days after surgery using anti-inflammatory drugs and cycloplegics to facilitate intracameral hemorrhage absorption.

Performing multiple surgical peripheral iridectomies is important to prevent peripheral anterior synechiae formation, decrease the chance for air-bubble or clot-induced acute angle closure glaucoma and reduce the chance for peripheral anterior synechiae formation and probable future chronic angle closure glaucoma. Sutures should be separate with tight and long bites. Due to severe thinning of recipient cornea in some areas, full-thickness suturing is sometimes unavoidable. Irregularity in the recipient-donor junction may lead to wound leakage; this may necessitate additional suturing. Care should be taken not to include iris stroma into the suture bites. Toxic suture reaction and cheese-wiring are common complications. Due to concomitant ocular surface disorders, small diameter corneal buttons are preferred. At least, 0.5mm graft disparity should be considered in all cases to ensure adequate anterior chamber depth. In the case of a heavy vascularized recipient cornea and compromised ocular surface, PKP or LKP may be considered as high risk. Therefore, in some cases using systemic immunosupression may be helpful for increasing donor cornea survival.

Keratolimbal Allograft Surgery (KLAL) and Living-related Conjunctival Limbal Allograft (lr-CLAL)

In the event of bilateral or unilateral total LSCD, transplantation of allogeneic limbal stem cells is the only remaining alternative for successful corneal surface restoration. This can be achieved by KLAL from cadaveric donors [87, 99] or by limbal-conjunctival allograft from living-related donors (lr-CLAL). [5, 99] A KLAL is a lamellar ring graft encompassing a minimal portion of scleral tissue, the entire limbus and the most peripheral portion of the cornea (Figures 9-A and 9-B). When compared with lr-CLAL, KLAL offers the advantages of providing stem cell supply because the entire eye limbal circumference is used for reconstruction, thus eliminating the concern of removing healthy limbal tissue from a normal eye, but still carrying the disadvantages of paucity of the conjunctival tissue for simultaneous conjunctival reconstruction. Although the short-term success rate of KLAL is comparable to those of CLAU, when the follow-up period is prolonged to more than 2 years, the success rate of KLAL dramatically drops to less than 60%. [32] This discrepancy is in great contrast to the overwhelmingly high success achieved by CLAU. One natural explanation for the failure of KLAL is allograft rejection because transplantation is carried out to the limbus, a highly vascularized area relatively abundant in Langerhans' cells. However, even under continuous systemic immunosuppression, the long-term results for KLAL over 3 years of follow-up remain unsatisfactory. [32] Autotransplantation of the limbus produces significantly better long-term outcomes compared to allogeneic limbal grafts from living-related and cadaveric donors. It has also been suggested that lr-CLAL fare better than KLAL. [131]

References

[1] Kenyon KR. Anatomy and pathology of the ocular surface. I*nt Ophthalmol Clin.* 1979 Summer;19(2):3-35.

[2] Friend J. Physiology of the conjunctiva: metabolism and biochemistry. In: Smolin G, Thoft RA, editors. *The Cornea: Scientific Foundation and Clinical Practice.* 2ed ed. Boston: Little, Brown; 1987. p. 52-62.

[3] Davanger M, Evensen A. Role of the pericorneal papillary structure in renewal of corneal epithelium. *Nature*. 1971 Feb 19;229(5286):560-1.

[4] Tseng SC. Regulation and clinical implications of corneal epithelial stem cells. *Mol Biol Rep.* 1996;23(1):47-58.

[5] Dua HS, Saini JS, Azuara-Blanco A, Gupta P. Limbal stem cell deficiency: concept, aetiology, clinical presentation, diagnosis and management. *Indian J Ophthalmol.* 2000 Jun;48(2):83-92.

[6] Lavker RM, Tseng SC, Sun TT. Corneal epithelial stem cells at the limbus: looking at some old problems from a new angle. *Exp Eye Res.* 2004 Mar;78(3):433-46.

[7] Schlotzer-Schrehardt U, Kruse FE. Identification and characterization of limbal stem cells. *Exp Eye Res.* 2005 Sep;81(3):247-64.

[8] Li W, Hayashida Y, Chen YT, Tseng SC. Niche regulation of corneal epithelial stem cells at the limbus. *Cell Res.* 2007 Jan;17(1):26-36.

[9] Liang L, Sheha H, Li J, Tseng SC. Limbal stem cell transplantation: new progresses and challenges. *Eye (Lond).* 2009 Oct;23(10):1946-53.

[10] Hatch KM, Dana R. The structure and function of the limbal stem cell and the disease states associated with limbal stem cell deficiency. *Int Ophthalmol Clin.* 2009 Winter;49(1):43-52.

[11] Buck RC. Measurement of centripetal migration of normal corneal epithelial cells in the mouse. *Invest Ophthalmol Vis Sci.* 1985 Sep;26(9):1296-9.

[12] Kinoshita S, Friend J, Thoft RA. Sex chromatin of donor corneal epithelium in rabbits. *Invest Ophthalmol Vis Sci.* 1981 Sep;21(3):434-41.

[13] Chen JJ, Tseng SC. Corneal epithelial wound healing in partial limbal deficiency. *Invest Ophthalmol Vis Sci.* 1990 Jul;31(7):1301-14.

[14] Chen JJ, Tseng SC. Abnormal corneal epithelial wound healing in partial-thickness removal of limbal epithelium. *Invest Ophthalmol Vis Sci.* 1991 Jul;32(8):2219-33.

[15] Friend J, Thoft RA. Functional competence of regenerating ocular surface epithelium. *Invest Ophthalmol Vis Sci.* 1978 Feb;17(2):134-9.

[16] Huang AJ, Tseng SC. Corneal epithelial wound healing in the absence of limbal epithelium. *Invest Ophthalmol Vis Sci.* 1991 Jan;32(1):96-105.

[17] Kruse FE, Chen JJ, Tsai RJ, Tseng SC. Conjunctival transdifferentiation is due to the incomplete removal of limbal basal epithelium. *Invest Ophthalmol Vis Sci.* 1990 Sep;31(9):1903-13.

[18] Thoft RA, Friend J. Biochemical transformation of regenerating ocular surface epithelium. *Invest Ophthalmol Vis Sci.* 1977 Jan;16(1):14-20.

[19] Thoft RA, Friend J, Murphy HS. Ocular surface epithelium and corneal vascularization in rabbits. I. T*he role of wounding. Invest Ophthalmol Vis Sci.* 1979 Jan;18(1):85-92.

[20] Kenyon KR. Morphology and pathologic responses of the cornea to disease. In: Smolin G, Thoft RA, editors. *The Cornea: Scientific Foundation and Clinical Practice.* 2ed ed. Boston: Little, Brown;; 1987. p. 63-98.

[21] Kenyon KR. Limbal autograft transplantation for chemical and thermal burns. *Dev Ophthalmol.* 1989;18:53-8.

[22] Tsai RJ, Sun TT, Tseng SC. Comparison of limbal and conjunctival autograft transplantation in corneal surface reconstruction in rabbits. *Ophthalmology.* 1990 Apr;97(4):446-55.

[23] Lee JH, Kenyon KR. Limbal Stem Cell Transplantation. *Contemporary Ophthalmology.* 2008;7(21):1-8.

[24] Thoft RA, Friend J. The X, Y, Z hypothesis of corneal epithelial maintenance. *Invest Ophthalmol Vis Sci.* 1983 Oct;24(10):1442-3.

[25] Park KS, Lim CH, Min BM, Lee JL, Chung HY, Joo CK, et al. The side population cells in the rabbit limbus sensitively increased in response to

the central cornea wounding. *Invest Ophthalmol Vis Sci.* 2006 Mar;47(3):892-900.

[26] Puangsricharern V, Tseng SC. Cytologic evidence of corneal diseases with limbal stem cell deficiency. *Ophthalmology.* 1995 Oct;102 (10):1476-85.

[27] Dua HS, Joseph A, Shanmuganathan VA, Jones RE. Stem cell differentiation and the effects of deficiency. *Eye* (Lond). 2003 Nov;17(8):877-85.

[28] Aitken D, Friend J, Thoft RA, Lee WR. An ultrastructural study of rabbit ocular surface transdifferentiation. *Invest Ophthalmol Vis Sci.* 1988 Feb;29(2):224-31.

[29] Li W, Chen YT, Hayashida Y, Blanco G, Kheirkah A, He H, et al. Down-regulation of Pax6 is associated with abnormal differentiation of corneal epithelial cells in severe ocular surface diseases. *J Pathol.* 2008 Jan;214(1):114-22.

[30] Pfister RR. Corneal stem cell disease: concepts, categorization, and treatment by auto- and homotransplantation of limbal stem cells. *CLAO J.* 1994 Jan;20(1):64-72.

[31] Holland EJ, Schwartz GS. Changing concepts in the management of severe ocular surface disease over twenty-five years. *Cornea.* 2000 Sep;19(5):688-98.

[32] Fernandes M, Sangwan VS, Rao SK, Basti S, Sridhar MS, Bansal AK, et al. Limbal stem cell transplantation. *Indian J Ophthalmol.* 2004 Mar;52(1):5-22.

[33] Dua HS, Azuara-Blanco A. Limbal stem cells of the corneal epithelium. *Surv Ophthalmol.* 2000 Mar-Apr;44(5):415-25.

[34] Dua HS, Forrester JV. The corneoscleral limbus in human corneal epithelial wound healing. *Am J Ophthalmol.* 1990 Dec 15;110(6):646-56.

[35] Schwartz GS, Holland EJ. Iatrogenic limbal stem cell deficiency. *Cornea.* 1998 Jan;17(1):31-7.

[36] Mackman G, Brightbill FS, Optiz JM. Corneal changes in aniridia. *Am J Ophthalmol.* 1979 Apr;87(4):497-502.

[37] Margo CE. Congenital aniridia: a histopathologic study of the anterior segment in children. *J Pediatr Ophthalmol Strabismus.* 1983 Sep-Oct;20(5):192-8.

[38] Nelson LB, Spaeth GL, Nowinski TS, Margo CE, Jackson L. Aniridia. A review. *Surv Ophthalmol.* 1984 May-Jun;28(6):621-42.

[39] Holland EJ. Epithelial transplantation for the management of severe ocular surface disease. *Trans Am Ophthalmol Soc.* 1996;94:677-743.

[40] Tseng SCG. Conjunctival grafting for corneal diseases. In: Tasman W, Jaeger EA, editors. *Duane's Clinical Ophthalmology.* Philadelphia: JB Lippincott; 1994. p. 1–11.

[41] Dua HS. The conjunctiva in corneal epithelial wound healing. *Br J Ophthalmol.* 1998 Dec;82(12):1407-11.

[42] Dua HS, Gomes JA, Singh A. Corneal epithelial wound healing. *Br J Ophthalmol.* 1994 May;78(5):401-8.

[43] Egbert PR, Lauber S, Maurice DM. A simple conjunctival biopsy. *Am J Ophthalmol.* 1977 Dec;84(6):798-801.

[44] Nishida K, Kinoshita S, Ohashi Y, Kuwayama Y, Yamamoto S. Ocular surface abnormalities in aniridia. *Am J Ophthalmol.* 1995 Sep; 120(3):368-75.

[45] Prabhasawat P, Tseng SC. Impression cytology study of epithelial phenotype of ocular surface reconstructed by preserved human amniotic membrane. *Arch Ophthalmol.* 1997 Nov;115(11):1360-7.

[46] Donisi PM, Rama P, Fasolo A, Ponzin D. Analysis of limbal stem cell deficiency by corneal impression cytology. *Cornea.* 2003 Aug;22(6):533-8.

[47] Sacchetti M, Lambiase A, Cortes M, Sgrulletta R, Bonini S, Merlo D. Clinical and cytological findings in limbal stem cell deficiency. *Graefes Arch Clin Exp Ophthalmol.* 2005 Sep;243(9):870-6.

[48] Fatima A, Iftekhar G, Sangwan VS, Vemuganti GK. Ocular surface changes in limbal stem cell deficiency caused by chemical injury: a histologic study of excised pannus from recipients of cultured corneal epithelium. *Eye (Lond).* 2008 Sep;22(9):1161-7.

[49] Dogru M, Tsubota K. Current concepts in ocular surface reconstruction. *Semin Ophthalmol.* 2005 Apr-Jun;20(2):75-93.

[50] Espana EM, Di Pascuale M, Grueterich M, Solomon A, Tseng SC. Keratolimbal allograft in corneal reconstruction. *Eye.* 2004 Apr;18(4):406-17.

[51] Holland EJ, Schwartz GS. The evolution of epithelial transplantation for severe ocular surface disease and a proposed classification system. *Cornea.* 1996 Nov;15(6):549-56.

[52] Terranova VP, Lyall RM. Chemotaxis of human gingival epithelial cells to laminin. A mechanism for epithelial cell apical migration. *J Periodontol.* 1986 May;57(5):311-7.

[53] Khodadoust AA, Silverstein AM, Kenyon DR, Dowling JE. Adhesion of regenerating corneal epithelium. The role of basement membrane. *Am J Ophthalmol.* 1968 Mar;65(3):339-48.

[54] Guo M, Grinnell F. Basement membrane and human epidermal differentiation in vitro. *J Invest Dermatol.* 1989 Sep;93(3):372-8.

[55] Tseng SC, Li DQ, Ma X. Suppression of transforming growth factor-beta isoforms, TGF-beta receptor type II, and myofibroblast differentiation in cultured human corneal and limbal fibroblasts by amniotic membrane matrix. *J Cell Physiol.* 1999 Jun;179(3):325-35.

[56] Tseng SC, Prabhasawat P, Barton K, Gray T, Meller D. Amniotic membrane transplantation with or without limbal allografts for corneal surface reconstruction in patients with limbal stem cell deficiency. *Arch Ophthalmol.* 1998 Apr;116(4):431-41.

[57] Holland EJ, Schwartz GS. The Paton lecture: Ocular surface transplantation: 10 years' experience. *Cornea.* 2004 Jul;23(5):425-31.

[58] Tsubota K, Satake Y, Ohyama M, Toda I, Takano Y, Ono M, et al. Surgical reconstruction of the ocular surface in advanced ocular cicatricial pemphigoid and Stevens-Johnson syndrome. *Am J Ophthalmol.* 1996 Jul;122(1):38-52.

[59] Shimazaki J, Yang HY, Tsubota K. Amniotic membrane transplantation for ocular surface reconstruction in patients with chemical and thermal burns. *Ophthalmology.* 1997 Dec;104(12):2068-76.

[60] Meallet MA, Espana EM, Grueterich M, Ti SE, Goto E, Tseng SC. Amniotic membrane transplantation with conjunctival limbal autograft for total limbal stem cell deficiency. *Ophthalmology.* 2003 Aug;110(8):1585-92.

[61] Kenyon KR, Tseng SC. Limbal autograft transplantation for ocular surface disorders. *Ophthalmology.* 1989 May;96(5):709-22; discussion 22-3.

[62] Nishiwaki-Dantas MC, Dantas PE, Reggi JR. Ipsilateral limbal translocation for treatment of partial limbal deficiency secondary to ocular alkali burn. *Br J Ophthalmol.* 2001 Sep;85(9):1031-3.

[63] Shimazaki J, Shinozaki N, Tsubota K. Transplantation of amniotic membrane and limbal autograft for patients with recurrent pterygium associated with symblepharon. *Br J Ophthalmol.* 1998 Mar;82(3):235-40.

[64] Tan DT, Ficker LA, Buckley RJ. *Limbal transplantation. Ophthalmology.* 1996 Jan;103(1):29-36.

[65] Basti S, Mathur U. Unusual intermediate-term outcome in three cases of limbal autograft transplantation. *Ophthalmology.* 1999 May;106(5):958-63.

[66] Rao SK, Rajagopal R, Sitalakshmi G, Padmanabhan P. Limbal autografting: comparison of results in the acute and chronic phases of ocular surface burns. *Cornea.* 1999 Mar;18(2):164-71.

[67] Sanghvi A, Basti S. Conjunctival transplantation for corneal surface reconstruction--case reports and review of literature. *Indian J Ophthalmol.* 1996 Mar;44(1):33-8.

[68] Tsai RJ, Tseng SC. Effect of stromal inflammation on the outcome of limbal transplantation for corneal surface reconstruction. *Cornea.* 1995 Sep;14(5):439-49.

[69] Moldovan SM, Borderie V, Baudrimont M, Laroche L. [Treatment of unilateral limbal stem cell deficiency syndrome by limbal autograft]. *J Fr Ophtalmol.* 1999 Apr;22(3):302-9.

[70] Tole DM, Edrich CL, Noble BA. Combined limbal and corneal autograft transplantation. *Eye (Lond).* 1999;13 (Pt 1):117-9.

[71] Cardoen L, Foets B. Limbal transplantation after chemical injuries of the eye. *Bull Soc Belge Ophtalmol.* 1999;272:105-10.

[72] Gatinel D, Nghiem MH, Chaine G. [Early limbal autograft after alkali burn of the ocular surface*]. J Fr Ophtalmol.* 1999 Feb;22(1):76-8.

[73] Frucht-Pery J, Siganos CS, Solomon A, Scheman L, Brautbar C, Zauberman H. Limbal cell autograft transplantation for severe ocular surface disorders. *Graefes Arch Clin Exp Ophthalmol.* 1998 Aug;236(8):582-7.

[74] Jenkins C, Tuft S, Liu C, Buckley R. Limbal transplantation in the management of chronic contact-lens-associated epitheliopathy. *Eye (Lond).* 1993;7 (Pt 5):629-33.

[75] Gerard M, Merle H, Chiambaretta F, Louis V, Richer R, Rigal D. [Surgical technique of limbal autotransplantation in severe and recent eye burns]. *J Fr Ophtalmol.* 1999 May;22(4):502-6.

[76] Mutlu FM, Sobaci G, Tatar T, Yildirim E. A comparative study of recurrent pterygium surgery: limbal conjunctival autograft transplantation versus mitomycin C with conjunctival flap. *Ophthalmology.* 1999 Apr;106(4):817-21.

[77] Rao SK, Lekha T, Mukesh BN, Sitalakshmi G, Padmanabhan P. Conjunctival-limbal autografts for primary and recurrent pterygia: technique and results. *Indian J Ophthalmol.* 1998 Dec;46(4):203-9.

[78] Kenyon KR, Wagoner MD, Hettinger ME. Conjunctival autograft transplantation for advanced and recurrent pterygium. *Ophthalmology.* 1985 Nov;92(11):1461-70.
[79] Koch JM, Mellin KB, Waubke TN. [The pterygium, Autologous conjunctiva-limbus transplantation as treatment]. *Ophthalmologe.* 1992 Apr;89(2):143-6.
[80] Guler M, Sobaci G, Ilker S, Ozturk F, Mutlu FM, Yildirim E. Limbal-conjunctival autograft transplantation in cases with recurrent pterygium. *Acta Ophthalmol (Copenh).* 1994 Dec;72(6):721-6.
[81] Shimazaki J, Yang HY, Tsubota K. Limbal autograft transplantation for recurrent and advanced pterygia. *Ophthalmic Surg Lasers.* 1996 Nov;27(11):917-23.
[82] Gris O, Guell JL, del Campo Z. Limbal-conjunctival autograft transplantation for the treatment of recurrent pterygium. *Ophthalmology.* 2000 Feb;107(2):270-3.
[83] Copeland RA, Jr., Char DH. Limbal autograft reconstruction after conjunctival squamous cell carcinoma. *Am J Ophthalmol.* 1990 Oct 15;110(4):412-5.
[84] Mashima Y, Yamada M, Yamada H. Limbal autograft transplantation for chronic ocular surface failures. *Jpn J Clin Ophthalmol.* 1993(47):607–10.
[85] Basti S, Rao SK. Current status of limbal conjunctival autograft. *Curr Opin Ophthalmol. 2000* Aug;11(4):224-32.
[86] Daya SM, Ilari FA. Living related conjunctival limbal allograft for the treatment of stem cell deficiency. *Ophthalmology.* 2001 Jan;108(1):126-33; discussion 33-4.
[87] Tsai RJ, Tseng SC. Human allograft limbal transplantation for corneal surface reconstruction. *Cornea.* 1994 Sep;13(5):389-400.
[88] Espana EM, Di Pascuale M, Grueterich M, Solomon A, Tseng SC. Keratolimbal allograft in corneal reconstruction. *Eye (Lond).* 2004 Apr;18(4):406-17.
[89] Schwab IR, Reyes M, Isseroff RR. Successful transplantation of bioengineered tissue replacements in patients with ocular surface disease. *Cornea.* 2000 Jul;19(4):421-6.
[90] Tsai RJ, Li LM, Chen JK. Reconstruction of damaged corneas by transplantation of autologous limbal epithelial cells. *N Engl J Med.* 2000 Jul 13;343(2):86-93.

[91] Grueterich M, Espana EM, Touhami A, Ti SE, Tseng SC. Phenotypic study of a case with successful transplantation of ex vivo expanded human limbal epithelium for unilateral total limbal stem cell deficiency. *Ophthalmology.* 2002 Aug;109(8):1547-52.

[92] Koizumi N, Inatomi T, Quantock AJ, Fullwood NJ, Dota A, Kinoshita S. Amniotic membrane as a substrate for cultivating limbal corneal epithelial cells for autologous transplantation in rabbits. *Cornea.* 2000 Jan;19(1):65-71.

[93] Koizumi N, Inatomi T, Suzuki T, Sotozono C, Kinoshita S. Cultivated corneal epithelial stem cell transplantation in ocular surface disorders. *Ophthalmology.* 2001 Sep;108(9):1569-74.

[94] Pellegrini G, Traverso CE, Franzi AT, Zingirian M, Cancedda R, De Luca M. Long-term restoration of damaged corneal surfaces with autologous cultivated corneal epithelium. *Lancet.* 1997 Apr 5;349(9057):990-3.

[95] Tseng SC, Di Pascuale MA, Liu DT, Gao YY, Baradaran-Rafii A. Intraoperative mitomycin C and amniotic membrane transplantation for fornix reconstruction in severe cicatricial ocular surface diseases. *Ophthalmology.* 2005 May;112(5):896-903.

[96] Kheirkhah A, Blanco G, Casas V, Hayashida Y, Raju VK, Tseng SC. Surgical strategies for fornix reconstruction based on symblepharon severity. *Am J Ophthalmol.* 2008 Aug;146(2):266-75.

[97] Akpek EK, Foster CS. Limbal stem-cell transplantation. *Int Ophthalmol Clin. 1*999 Winter;39(1):71-82.

[98] Holland EJ, Croasdale CR. Epithelial transplantation for management of severe ocular surface disease. In: Brightbill FS, editor. *Corneal Surgery: Theory, Technique and Tissue.* 3rd ed. St. Louis: Mosby; 1999. p. 488-99.

[99] Dua HS, Azuara-Blanco A. Allo-limbal transplantation in patients with limbal stem cell deficiency. *Br J Ophthalmol.* 1999 Apr;83(4):414-9.

[100] Samson CM, Nduaguba C, Baltatzis S, Foster CS. Limbal stem cell transplantation in chronic inflammatory eye disease. *Ophthalmology.* 2002 May;109(5):862-8.

[101] Santos MS, Gomes JA, Hofling-Lima AL, Rizzo LV, Romano AC, Belfort R, Jr. Survival analysis of conjunctival limbal grafts and amniotic membrane transplantation in eyes with total limbal stem cell deficiency. *Am J Ophthalmol.* 2005 Aug;140(2):223-30.

[102] Dua HS, Azuara-Blanco A. Autologous limbal transplantation in patients with unilateral corneal stem cell deficiency. *Br J Ophthalmol.* 2000 Mar;84(3):273-8.

[103] Ivekovic R, Tedeschi-Reiner E, Novak-Laus K, Andrijevic-Derk B, Cima I, Mandic Z. Limbal graft and/or amniotic membrane transplantation in the treatment of ocular burns. *Ophthalmologica.* 2005 Sep-Oct;219(5):297-302.

[104] Kheirkhah A, Raju VK, Tseng SC. Minimal conjunctival limbal autograft for total limbal stem cell deficiency. *Cornea.* 2008 Jul;27(6):730-3.

[105] Williams KA, Brereton HM, Aggarwal R, Sykes PJ, Turner DR, Russ GR, et al. Use of DNA polymorphisms and the polymerase chain reaction to examine the survival of a human limbal stem cell allograft. *Am J Ophthalmol.* 1995 Sep;120(3):342-50.

[106] Solomon A, Ellies P, Anderson DF, Touhami A, Grueterich M, Espana EM, et al. Long-term outcome of keratolimbal allograft with or without penetrating keratoplasty for total limbal stem cell deficiency. *Ophthalmology.* 2002 Jun;109(6):1159-66.

[107] Cauchi PA, Ang GS, Azuara-Blanco A, Burr JM. A systematic literature review of surgical interventions for limbal stem cell deficiency in humans. *Am J Ophthalmol.* 2008 Aug;146(2):251-9.

[108] Sangwan VS. Limbal stem cells in health and disease. *Biosci Rep.* 2001 Aug;21(4):385-405.

[109] Shimazaki J, Kosaka K, Shimmura S, Tsubota K. Amniotic membrane transplantation with conjunctival autograft for recurrent pterygium. *Ophthalmology.* 2003 Jan;110(1):119-24.

[110] Akinci A, Zilelioglu O. Comparison of limbal-conjunctival autograft and intraoperative 0.02% mitomycin-C for treatment of primary pterygium. *Int Ophthalmol.* 2007 Oct;27(5):281-5.

[111] Al Fayez MF. Limbal versus conjunctival autograft transplantation for advanced and recurrent pterygium. *Ophthalmology.* 2002 Sep;109(9):1752-5.

[112] Biswas MC, Shaw C, Mandal R, Islam MN, Chakroborty M. Treatment of pterygium with conjunctival limbal autograft and mitomycin C--a comparative study. *J Indian Med Assoc.* 2007 Apr;105(4):200, 2, 4.

[113] Fallah MR, Golabdar MR, Amozadeh J, Zare MA, Moghimi S, Fakhraee G. Transplantation of conjunctival limbal autograft and amniotic

membrane vs mitomycin C and amniotic membrane in treatment of recurrent pterygium. *Eye (Lond).* 2008 Mar;22(3):420-4.

[114] Kilic A, Gurler B. The efficiency of limbal conjunctival autografting in pterygium surgery. *Eur J Ophthalmol.* 2006 May-Jun;16(3):365-70.

[115] Shimazaki J, Shimmura S, Fujishima H, Tsubota K. Association of preoperative tear function with surgical outcome in severe Stevens-Johnson syndrome. *Ophthalmology.* 2000 Aug;107(8):1518-23.

[116] Tsubota K, Satake Y, Kaido M, Shinozaki N, Shimmura S, Bissen-Miyajima H, et al. Treatment of severe ocular-surface disorders with corneal epithelial stem-cell transplantation. *N Engl J Med.* 1999 Jun 3;340(22):1697-703.

[117] Tsubota K, Toda I, Saito H, Shinozaki N, Shimazaki J. Reconstruction of the corneal epithelium by limbal allograft transplantation for severe ocular surface disorders. *Ophthalmology.* 1995 Oct;102(10):1486-96.

[118] Meller D, Pires RT, Mack RJ, Figueiredo F, Heiligenhaus A, Park WC, et al. Amniotic membrane transplantation for acute chemical or thermal burns. *Ophthalmology.* 2000 May;107(5):980-9; discussion 90.

[119] John T, Foulks GN, John ME, Cheng K, Hu D. Amniotic membrane in the surgical management of acute toxic epidermal necrolysis. *Ophthalmology.* 2002 Feb;109(2):351-60.

[120] Kim JC, Tseng SC. Transplantation of preserved human amniotic membrane for surface reconstruction in severely damaged rabbit corneas. *Cornea.* 1995 Sep;14(5):473-84.

[121] Chang MA, Chuck RS. Total anterior corneal surface and epithelial stem cell harvesting: current microkeratomes and beyond. *Expert Rev Med Devices.* 2004 Nov;1(2):251-8.

[122] Kwitko S, Marinho D, Barcaro S, Bocaccio F, Rymer S, Fernandes S, et al. Allograft conjunctival transplantation for bilateral ocular surface disorders. *Ophthalmology.* 1995 Jul;102(7):1020-5.

[123] Rao SK, Rajagopal R, Sitalakshmi G, Padmanabhan P. Limbal allografting from related live donors for corneal surface reconstruction. *Ophthalmology.* 1999 Apr;106(4):822-8.

[124] Morgan S, Murray A. Limbal autotransplantation in the acute and chronic phases of severe chemical injuries. *Eye (Lond).* 1996;10 (Pt 3):349-54.

[125] Kim JY, Djalilian AR, Schwartz GS, Holland EJ. Ocular surface reconstruction: limbal stem cell transplantation. *Ophthalmol Clin North Am.* 2003 Mar;16(1):67-77.

[126] Baradaran-Rafii A, Ebrahimi M, Kanavi MR, Taghi-Abadi E, Aghdami N, Eslani M, et al. Midterm outcomes of autologous cultivated limbal stem cell transplantation with or without penetrating keratoplasty. *Cornea.* 2010 May;29(5):502-9.

[127] Higa K, Shimazaki J. Recent advances in cultivated epithelial transplantation. *Cornea.* 2008 Sep;27 Suppl 1:S41-7.

[128] Shortt AJ, Secker GA, Notara MD, Limb GA, Khaw PT, Tuft SJ, et al. Transplantation of ex vivo cultured limbal epithelial stem cells: a review of techniques and clinical results. *Surv Ophthalmol.* 2007 Sep-Oct;52(5):483-502.

[129] Miri A, Al-Deiri B, Dua HS. Long-term outcomes of autolimbal and allolimbal transplants. *Ophthalmology.* Jun;117(6):1207-13.

[130] Miri A, Al-Deiri B, Dua HS. Long-term Outcomes of Autolimbal and Allolimbal Transplants. *ophthalmology.* 2010.

[131] Wylegala E, Dobrowolski D, Tarnawska D, Janiszewska D, Gabryel B, Malecki A, et al. Limbal stem cells transplantation in the reconstruction of the ocular surface: 6 years experience. *Eur J Ophthalmol.* 2008 Nov-Dec;18(6):886-90.

In: Advances in Eye Research. Volume 1 ISBN 978-1-61324-169-1
Editor: William L. Thomsen, pp. 47-63

Chapter II

Gene Therapy for Corneal Diseases

Ashish Tandon[1,2], *Jonathan C. K. Tovey*[1,2], *Ajay Sharma*[1,2], *and Rajiv R. Mohan*[1,2,3,*]

[1]Harry S. Truman Memorial Veterans' Hospital, Columbia, MO 65201, [2]Mason Eye Institute, School of Medicine, University of Missouri, Columbia, Missouri 65212, and [3]College of Veterinary Medicine, University of Missouri-Columbia, Columbia, Missouri 65211, USA

Abstract

The World Health Organization estimates that 45 million people worldwide are suffering from blindness. Corneal and other ocular surface diseases are the 3rd leading cause of global blindness. Conventional treatments are effective but associated with significant side effects that can undermine their clinical utility. Gene therapy is an emerging innovative technology for eye disease treatment and prevention. The successful restoration of vision in a few human patients outlines its enormous potential in treating eye disorders. Gene therapy may

[*] Corresponding author: Rajiv R. Mohan, Ph.D.; Associate Professor, Mason Eye Institute, School of Medicine, University of Missouri-Columbia. 1 Hospital Drive, Columbia, MO 65212; Ph (573) 884-1449, Fax (573) 814-6551; E-mail: mohanr@health.missouri.edu

potentially treat genetic and acquired corneal blindness due to scarring, graft rejection, angiogenesis, dystrophies, keratitis, Sjogren syndrome, and ocular surface disorders. Gene therapy entails the use of novel vectors to transfer therapeutic genes into corneal cells to modulate the expression of a particular protein, growth factor, or cytokine that in turn will modify corneal disease. Two major determinants for the success of gene therapy are the use of an appropriate vector and gene delivery technique. Numerous viral vectors such as adenovirus, adeno-associated virus (AAV), lentivirus, and retrovirus, as well as nonviral vectors such as lipid, gold nanopariticle, dendrimer and different catatropic polymers have been tested for ocular diseases. Each of these vectors has its own advantages and limitations. Recently, next generation AAV vectors were developed by creating a point mutation that increased transgene delivery into the retina 15-30 fold at 10 fold less doses. Our ongoing studies with these next generation mutant AAV vectors and gold nanopariticle nonviral vectors suggest that these delivery systems are 10-25 fold more efficient than conventional viral and nonviral vectors for delivering genes in the cornea in animal experimental models.

Introduction

Human gene therapy is one of the most exciting fields in biomedical research. Gene therapy is defined as an experimental treatment to cure or ultimately prevent a disease by either replacing defective mutant genes with new functional genes or entirely changing the expression of an individual's genes. This approach may eventually be adopted for many diseases like hemophilia, Parkinson's disease, acquired immune deficiency syndrome (AIDS), cancer, severe combined immunodeficiency (SCID), and ocular surface disorders. Friedmann and Roblin first proposed the concept of gene therapy in 1972, but to date clinical applications remain few and far between due to inefficient delivery of therapeutic genes in the target tissue (Friedmann and Roblin, 1972). September 14th, 1990 marked the first use of gene therapy in humans when Ashanti DeSilva was treated for SCID with the treatment working for a few months. Although gene therapy technology is still in its adolescence, it has been used with some success.

In the eye, gene therapy is a novel approach to treat genetic and acquired disorders especially on the ocular surface. The recent success of restoring vision with gene therapy in patients with Leber's congenital amaurosis reaffirms the potential of this form of molecular medicine to treat eye diseases.

This has encouraged many more ocular gene therapy clinical trials around the world including the United States. Nonetheless, the US Food and Drug Administration has not yet granted approval for treating patients with gene therapy. The completion of the human genome project has provided rich information about genes involved in various biological and pathological processes significantly enhancing the scope of gene therapy to cure blindness. This chapter provides an overview of ocular surface gene transfer studies performed by our laboratory and other investigators.

2. Gene Therapy Methods for the Cornea

A transparent cornea is essential for normal vision. The cornea is composed of five layers from anterior to posterior; epithelium, Bowman's layer, stroma, Descemet's membrane, and endothelium. Corneal tissue is particularly suited for gene therapy because of its accessibility as the outermost layer of the eye. In addition, the cornea enjoys an immune-privileged status as one of the few organs isolated from the general circulatory and immune systems. Furthermore, repeated application of vector and visual monitoring can be carried out with relative ease. These characteristics render the cornea ideal in testing gene therapy to treat corneal disorders such as corneal neovascularization, corneal scarring, corneal graft rejection, and monogenic lysosomal storage disorders like mucopolysaccharidosis VI and VII syndrome.

The success of gene therapy largely depends on vectors, which play an important role in introducing foreign genes into cells. In fact, vectors and vector-delivery technique are the two chief determinants of successful treatment with gene therapy. The efficiency of numerous vectors and vector-delivery techniques for delivering genes to the ocular surface has been evaluated employing *in vitro*, *in vivo* or *ex vivo* models. Each vector has its own advantages and limitations. A brief description of various gene therapy vectors is discussed below:

2.1. Viral Vectors

Viruses are nucleoproteins that attack target (host) cells in order to replicate. Once inside the cell, viral RNA or DNA is incorporated into the cell's own protein synthesis, resulting in production of viral copies.This characteristic of viruses has been exploited for gene therapy. Among viral vectors, recombinant adenovirus, adeno-associated virus (AAV), retrovirus, and lentivirus have been found to efficiently transport genes in the cornea.

Adenovirus

Adenoviruses are non-enveloped icosaherdral particles composed of nucleocapsid and double stranded DNA. Adenoviruses, the first viral vectors used in the ocular surface, are the most popular vectors for corneal gene therapy as they offer several advantages. These vectors are capable of transducing dividing as well as non dividing cells. This is a great benefit as the cornea contains actively dividing epithelial cells as well as non dividing endothelial cells and quiescent stromal keratocytes which are known to undergo mitosis during pathologic conditions. Adenoviruses, like most vectors, have some undesirable features. These include the induction of a pro-inflammatory response and a short term transgene expression due to the fact that they integrate into the host genome. Literary reports reveal that these vectors have failed to transfer genes in rat, sheep, and rabbit corneal epithelium. The Qi group studied the effect of adenoviral vector-mediated glial cell-derived gene delivery on the survival of primary human corneal epithelial cells *in vitro*. They found that this neurotrophic factor is a survival growth factor for cultured human corneal epithelium (Qi et al., 2008). However, adenoviruses have shown the best transduction efficiency for corneal endothelial cells in comparison to vectors developed from equine, lenti, or bacullovirus. The human corneal endothelium has a unique advantage as a target for gene therapy because it is a monolayer of cells on the internal surface of the cornea with a well-defined anatomy (Oral et al., 1997).

Several investigators have shown that recombinant adenovirus-mediated soluble VEGF receptor sFlk-1 expression in the cornea inhibits the development of corneal neovascularization supporting the idea that adenoviral vectors are capable of high-level transgene expression. Recently recombinant adenovirus-driven c-met overexpression in human organ-cultured corneas was tested for correction of diabetic abnormalities. Results demonstrated that this recombinant adenovirus may restore HGF signaling, normalize diabetic marker patterns, and accelerate wound healing (Saghizadeh et al., 2010). In glaucoma filtration surgery, Yang et al., (2009) constructed an adenovirus recombinant vector Ad-p27 and administered it in the eye through the subconjunctiva in a rabbit model. They found that p27(KIP1) is a potential adjunctive agent for inhibition of wound healing after filtration surgery (Yang et al., 2009).

Retrovirus

Retroviruses are enveloped RNA viruses belonging to the family retroviridae. This virion is cone-shaped, 80-100 nm in size, and contains two copies of 7-11 kb single-stranded RNA genomes complexed with nucleocapsid protein. The retrovirus genome typically contains four genes *gag*, *pro*, *pol* and *env* flanked by long terminal repeats (LTR's) at both ends. All four genes are characterized by their functions. The *gag* gene is responsible for capsid, matrix, and nucleocapsid proteins while *pro* encodes the enzyme protease. The *pol* gene encodes reverse transcriptase as well as integrase while the env gene is responsible for envelop proteins. Retroviruses transduce cells through an interaction between viral envelope proteins and a cell surface receptor.

The principal advantage of retroviral vectors is their ability to integrate into the host genome and thus provide long-term stable transgene expression. They also have low immunogenic potential and a wide spectrum of cell tropism. Additionally, these vectors can accommodate large DNA inserts up to 8 kb and can generate relatively high titers (10^6-10^7 cfu/ml). These attributes increase the usefulness of these vectors. Retroviruses unfortunately are not without fault. Like adenoviruses, the main limitation of retroviruses is that they lack the capacity to transform non-dividing cells.

In the ocular surface, many investigators have demonstrated the use of retroviral vectors. However, retroviral vectors have not been evaluated to a large extent for delivering genes in the cornea *in vivo*. Seitz and colleagues used this vector on cultured human and rabbit corneal fibroblasts and showed low levels of transgene transduction. They also found that addition of polycations significantly increased transduction efficiency of the retrovirus vector (Seitz et al., 1998). Later they reported much improved transduction efficiency of retroviral vectors for delivering transgene in human and rabbit fibroblasts *in vitro* (Seitz et al., 1998a). Another finding of this study was that human corneal cells had higher susceptibility for retrovirus transduction than rabbit keratocytes. It was reported that retrovirus vector can successfully transduce up to 40% of keratocytes in laser ablated rabbit corneas *in vivo* (Seitz et al., 1998a).

Another study showed that retroviral vectors can effectively transduce corneal epithelial progenitor cells and express transgene for a long duration in the cornea *in vitro* and *in vivo* (Bradshaw et al., 1999). These studies not only exhibited the efficacy of retrovirus as a vector but also highlited the potential of gene therapy to treat corneal diseases. However, the advent of lentivirus vectors reduced the popularity of retroviral vectors for corneal gene therapy.

Lentiviral Vectors

Lentiviruses are spherical RNA viruses belonging to the lentivirinae genus and retroviridae family. Lentiviruses vary in size from approximately 80-100 nm and consist of a 9.2 kb genome. Lentiviruses, unlike adenoviruses, cause low inflammation and immunogenicity, produce long term gene expression, and transduce genes in noncycling cells. Disabled lentiviral vectors are a good candidate for corneal gene therapy as they can deliver therapeutic genes in non- or slow-dividing corneal cells such as keratocytes and endothelial cells. Many studies have demonstrated transgene expression in ocular tissue following transduction with lentiviruses. The use of lentiviruses in prolonged rodent corneal allograft survival and *ex vivo* use in transduction of the donor cornea has also been reported. For allograft survival, Parker and associates recently compared interleukins in adenoviruses and lentiviruses (Parker et al., 2010). Due to their long-term expression, these disabled lentivirus vectors have been used to deliver large genes to all the three major layers of the human cornea *in vitro* as well as in mouse corneal endothelium *in vivo*. Recently, to overcome the problem of graft rejection, *ex vivo* gene therapy of the donor cornea was performed and showed that recombinant lentiviruses are helpful in modulating graft failure in experimental models. New procedures using a femtosecond laser for gene transfer into the stroma of pig corneas for the delivery of therapeutic factors to treat or prevent recurrent corneal angiogenesis were recently employed using human immunodeficiency virus (HIV)1-derived lentiviral vector expressing green fluorescent protein (GFP). Previously, using lentivirus vector and topical application or microinjection, our research group delivered enhanced GFP genes into mouse corneal stroma following epithelium removal (Figure 1). The results supported our hypothesis that gene delivery in the cornea is regulated by both vector and vector-delivery techniques and not by vector alone. Lentivirus-mediated gene delivery did not show toxic effects suggesting the vector may be appropriate for gene therapy-based treatment in human patients. However, safety remains a major concern for using lentivirus vectors, since they originate from HIV.

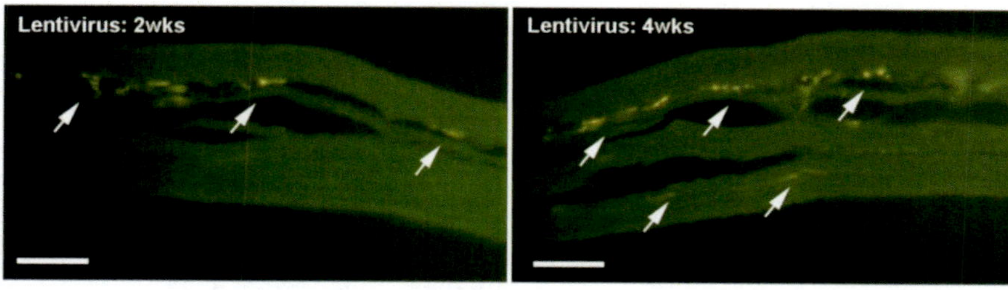

Figure 1. Lentivirus mediated enhanced green fluorescent gene delivery in the mouse corneal stroma. Vector was applied topically for two minutes on the cornea after removing corneal epithelium with #64 beaver surgical blade. Transgene delivery in the cornea was examined two weeks (left panel) and four weeks (right panel) following vector application. Scale bar denotes 50 microns.

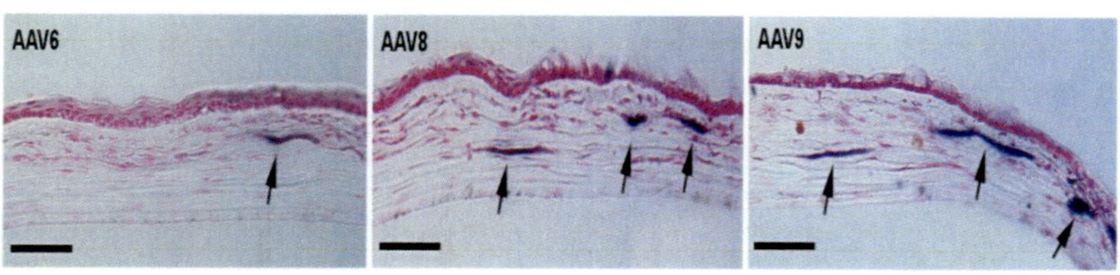

Figure 2. Effect of AAV serotype on level of gene delivery in mouse cornea, *in vivo*. AAV serotype 6, 8, and 9 vectors containing alkaline phosphatase marker gene showed varied expression. Vectors were applied topically on de-epithelialized mouse cornea for two minutes. AAV serotypes 8 (middle panel) and AAV9 (right panel) showed significantly higher transgene delivery compared to AAV6 (left panel). Scale bar denotes 50 microns.

Adeno-associated Virus

Recombinant adeno-associated virus (AAV) is a small nonpathogenic, replication-defective, 4.7 kb DNA virus that belongs to the Parvovirus family under the Dependovirus genus. Among the various tested viral vectors, AAV is a more popular vector for ocular gene therapy. Because of its properties, AAV has been used in many preclinical and clinical studies of various eye diseases. AAV vectors are currently among the most frequently used viral vectors for gene therapy due to their lack of apparent pathogenicity, their capability of producing long term gene expression, and their ability to infect both dividing and non-dividing cells. Although AAV seems like the perfect delivery shuttle, it too has a shortcoming. The main drawback of this vector is that the maximal capacity of carried DNA is only 4.7 kb.

These attributes provide an all but favorable alternative for delivering genes into keratocytes and corneal endothelial cells. However, to date limited studies have been performed to evaluate the characteristics, mode of action, and utility of these vectors for corneal gene therapy.

Although more than 100 AAV serotypes have been isolated from humans and other primates, only AAV serotypes 1-9 (AAV1-9) have been used to generate vectors for gene delivery in ocular and non-ocular tissues. AAV is a promising vector for corneal gene therapy but technical difficulties in preparing high titers of AAV pose a challenge for general use and clinical application. Mohan and cohorts for the first time defined efficient methods for *in situ* transgene delivery into keratocytes of the rabbit cornea with AAV2 using lamellar flap techniques (Mohan et al., 2003). Later studies from the same group compared the transduction efficiency of various AAV serotypes for delivering genes in the cornea using *in vitro* and *in vivo* models. AAV5 was found to be more efficient in delivering genes in the rabbit cornea compared to AAV2 (Mohan et al., 2005a). Among AAV6, AAV8, and AAV9 vectors, AAV8 and AAV9 showed high transduction compared to AAV6 in the mouse stroma as evident from Figure 2 (Sharma et al., 2010a). Interestingly, this study also revealed that AAV serotypes could have different transduction efficiencies for corneal cells grown in culture and *in vivo* (Sharma et al., 2010a and Sharma et al., 2010b). For example, AAV6 transduced large populations of keratocytes grown in culture from donor human corneas but transduced few keratocytes in the mouse cornea *in vivo* (Figure 3). Thus, it is important to examine the efficacy of different AAV serotypes for corneal gene therapy in various animal models.

Of late, several hybrid AAV vectors have been engineered using the genome of AAV serotype 2 and the capsid protein of AAV serotypes 1-9 for gene therapy. The newly produced hybrid AAV vectors have shown improved trangene delivery in many tissues including the eye. However, apart from the AAV5 vector, the transduction efficiency of other newly developed hybrid AAV vectors for the cornea has not been investigated. Recently our laboratory tested the cellular tropism and relative transduction efficiency of AAV2/6, AAV2/8 and AAV2/9 vectors for the cornea using primary cultures of human corneal fibroblasts. We found that the different AAV serotypes tested do not induce significant cell death and are safe for corneal gene therapy (Sharma et al., 2010b). We also showed the cellular tropism and relative transduction efficiency of three AAV serotypes, AAV6, AAV8, and AAV9 for corneal gene delivery using mouse cornea *in vivo* and donor human cornea *ex vivo*. Viral vector was applied topically onto mouse cornea *in vivo* and human cornea *ex vivo* after removing the epithelium. Mouse corneas were harvested at three different time points 4, 14, and 30 days while human corneas were processed at day 5 after AAV vector application. The analysis of this data reaffirmed that AAV vectors are efficient and safe for corneal gene therapy (Sharma et al., 2010b).

2.2. Non-viral Methods

Introduction of plasmid DNA expressing therapeutic genes into target cells without a viral vector has many advantages for treating corneal diseases. Non-viral gene therapy is much safer compared to viral gene therapy because of its non-toxic, non-pathogenic, and non-immunogenic nature. Furthermore, the commercial production of plasmid DNA is relatively simple, nonhazardous, and cost effective. Nevertheless, low transfection efficiency makes non-viral gene therapy less popular. The application of naked plasmid on target cells alone can deliver small amounts of DNA but usually it is insufficient to provide therapeutic levels of transgene expression in host cells. In order to enhance the amount of plasmid delivery into cells many strategies including a variety of techniques, chemicals, and more recently nanoparticles, have been introduced.

Techniques such as microinjection, gene gun (ballistic transfer), electroporation, sonoporation, hydrodynamic method, laser irradiation, iontophoresis, dendrimer, nanoparticle mediated, as well as peptide targeting are classified as physical methods of DNA delivery. All these methods use unmodified plasmid DNA for gene delivery. Beside these, the femetosecond laser has been used recently to introduce viral vectors carrying a reporter gene by creating a corneal stromal pocket (Bemelmans et al., 2009). Topical application of direct naked plasmid DNA into the corneal stroma to prevent herpetic eye disease and corneal neovascularization has been described by many experimenters. Stromal hydration and filtration bleb surgery procedures are among the surgical approaches that have been employed for *in vivo* gene delivery into corneal tissue.

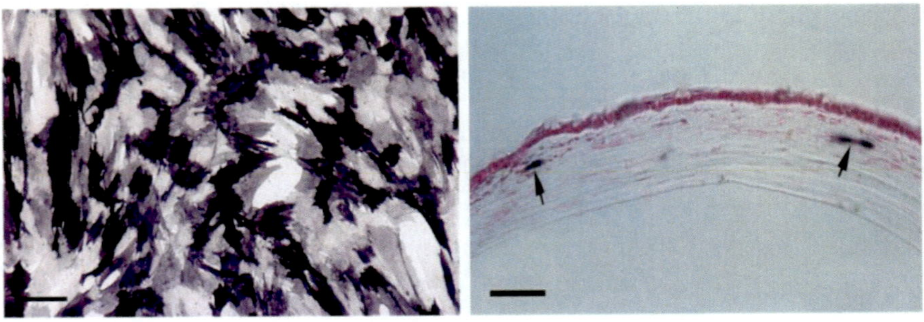

Figure 3. AAV serotype 6 showed vastly different transduction efficiency for corneal stroma *in vitro* and *in vivo*. An exceptionally high transgene (alkaline phosphatase) delivery was detected in human corneal keratocyte cultures treated with AAV6 (left panel) whereas mouse cornea treated with AAV6 transduced few keratocytes *in vivo* (right panel). Left panel scale bar denotes 200 microns. Right panel scale bar denotes 50 microns.

In the ballistic transfer/gene gun method, plasmid DNA was mixed with cDNA-coated gold microparticles and delivered into target tissues using the force generated by the gun. Several investigators have reported successful administration of plasmid DNA into rabbit as well as mouse cornea via the gene gun method (Wang et al., 2002). However this method has multiple side effects such as destruction of epithelial morphology, injury to stroma, ocular surface irritation, etc. (Mohan et al., 2005). Some studies have also reported cell nuclei damage in the corneal endothelium after gene gun utilization.

Electroporation and iontophoresis mainly refers to the use of electric current to deliver naked circular DNA into cell cultures. Although several hypotheses have been put forth to explain the mechanism of electroporation, it is still unclear. The most plausible mechanisms are the permeabilization of cell membrane and electro-osmotic effect. Oshima pioneered the electroporation technique to transfer genes in corneal endothelium (Oshima et al., 1998). The Oshima group later described successful gene transfer in corneal stroma using the same techniques (Oshima et al., 2002). A major advantage of this method over viral technology was that it provided rapid transgene expression in the ocular surface *in vivo*. The disadvantage of electroporation is that higher electric current that increased transgene delivery was associated with corneal damage.

Dendrimers are repeatedly branched, roughly spherical, large molecules having three major portions. These include a core, an inner shell, and an outer shell that can encapsulate various molecules including plasmid DNA. Hudde et al. (1999) were the first to use activated polyamidoamine dendrimers for gene transfer into the corneal endothelium. The result of their study shows that this approach can be beneficial in corneal allograft rejection or in the treatment of other disorders of the corneal endothelium. Cationic liposome based formulations have also been used by different researchers for the transduction of plasmid DNA in corneal endothelial cells (Pleyer et al., 2001, and Klebe et al., 2001). These studies aimed to determine the efficiency and toxicity of liposome-mediated gene transfer in corneal endothelial cells.

The National Institutes of Health has defined materials less than 100 nm in size as nanoparticles. The dawn of nanotechnology has provided a large pool of nanoparticles as potential vectors for drug and gene delivery. The nanoparticles (NPs) that are used currently in eye research include polymeric (PEI, poly-L-lysine, PLGA or PLA) or hybrid (metallic-polymeric) NPs, PEG-substituted-30mer lysine, PLGA NPs, DOTAP polymeric nanoparticles and PEI stabilized gold nanoparticles. Different studies reveal this gold nanoparticle approach as holding great potential in the treatment of diseases including corneal neovascularization.

Other methods that have been used recently for ocular gene therapy include a synthetic peptide vector system (Collins et al., 2004), a novel bubble liposome and ultrasound mediated gene transfer method (Yamashita et al., 2007), and a hyaluronic acid-chitosan nanoparticle (de la Fuente et al., 2008).

3. Application of Gene Therapy for Corneal Diseases

Gene therapy of the ocular surface has the potential to treat and cure inherited and acquired ocular disorders and metabolic diseases affecting the cornea. Researchers in the corneal gene therapy field have chiefly concentrated on different acquired ocular disorders such as corneal graft rejection, corneal wound healing, alkali burn, corneal scarring, corneal dystrophies, and corneal neovascularization.

3.1. Corneal Graft Rejection and Corneal Transplantation

Corneal transplantation is an increasingly common procedure to address many potentially blinding ocular diseases. Approximately 40,000 transplants in the United States are performed every year. The success rate of corneal transplantation varies from 60-75%. Even though the cornea's immune-priviledged status confers a strong protective factor, the main cause of corneal transplant failure is immunological rejection/graft rejection. The risk factors for graft rejection include neovascularization, inflammation, glaucoma, and a history of previous graft rejection.

Many gene therapy studies have been conducted for prevention of corneal graft rejection. Earlier studies report that cytotoxic T-lymphocytes stimulate a cascade of events that leads to graft destruction. Many researchers are focused on the use and efficacy of cytotoxic T-lymphocyte-associated antigen-4 conjugated to the heavy chain of IgG (CTLA-4 Ig) in gene therapy to control graft rejection. It is also thought that damage to the endothelium is crucial during this process. Another factor that plays an important role in corneal graft survival versus rejection is cytokines. During graft rejection, the elevated levels of proinflammatory cytokines such as T helper (Th) cell type-1 have been detected in corneal tissues as well as the anterior chamber. Th type-2 cytokines like interleukin 10 (IL10) and IL4 on the other hand show reciprocal (inhibitory) effect in comparison to Th1 cytokines. This proinflammatory vs inhibitory battle between Th type-1 and Th type-2 cytokines has been the focus of many gene therapy studies on graft survival (Mohan et al., 2005).

3.2. Corneal Scarring (Haze)

Corneal scarring is a term used to depict corneal opacity caused by excimer laser techniques like photorefractive keratectomy (PRK) surgery, particularly in patients undergoing high myopia correction. The basic phenomenon behind the cause of corneal scarring is the transformation of stromal keratocytes into activated fibroblasts that proliferate and migrate to the anterior stromal compartment where they synthesize new disorganized collagen and aberrant extracellular matrix (ECM) that leads to opacity. The current treatment of corneal scarring is mitomycin-C which mainly induces the apoptosis of stromal keratocytes and prevents corneal scarring. Many studies reveal that there is a need of additional therapies for the treatment of corneal scarring due to the side effect of mitomycin-C. Gene therapy offers a unique approach for intercepting the molecular events involved in the development of corneal haze. The different gene therapy approaches that may prove useful in the treatment of corneal haze include blockage of keratocyte proliferation, blockade of cyclins and cyclin-dependent kinases for controlling cell division, and apoptosis of activated keratocytes.

3.3. Corneal Neovascularization (CNV)

Avascularity is vital for the cornea to remain transparent. Several factors are responsible for corneal neovascularization (CNV). These include infection, degenerative disease, physical and chemical damage, mechanical and surgical injury, and immunological diseases. CNV affects more than 1.4 million Americans every year and plays a pivotal role in the inflammation responsible for corneal graft rejection. For the treatment of CNV various antimicrobial, anti-inflammatory as well as immunosuppressant drugs may be used depending on the etiology of CNV.

Various studies hold that vascular endothelial growth factor (VEGF) plays a key role in neovascularization. A range of vectors and gene therapy strategies have been developed and examined to suppress VEGF-induced corneal angiogenesis using experimental models. The genes that have been used in different studies include Flt-1 (VEGF receptor 1) and plasmid encoding for specific VEGF binding domains of soluble Flt-1 namely Flt23K, or Flt24K peptides. Many investigators have shown that these peptides are not released outside the cell and hence are capable of neutralizing intracellular VEGF. Other reports show that lentivirus-mediated delivery of endostatin and kringle-5 domain of plasminogen fusion protein inhibits CNV. Angiostatin is another potent, recently identified anti-angiogenic agent that has effectively reduced alkali-induced CNV in rabbit cornea. Topical applications of cytokines like IL12 or IL10 also have shown marked suppression of CNV.

3.4. Corneal Dystrophies

Corneal gene therapy approaches can also address the problem of corneal dystrophies. However, the lack of an appropriate model limits the development of new treatment. There are many types of corneal dystrophies, the main ones being hereditary endothelial dystrophy, mucopolysaccharidosis, Fuch's dystrophy, and posterior polymorphous dystrophy. Preliminary work has been reported and suggests that keratoconus, iridocorneal, as well as Behcet's disease of the cornea may be potential candidates for gene therapy. Very few gene transfer studies using corneal buttons collected from patients or rodent models have been performed to evaluate the efficacy of gene therapy in corneal dystrophies. Recently in type VII mucopolysaccharidosis, adenovirus vector encoding human beta-glucuronidase gene was applied in the anterior chamber to deliver transgene to corneal cells. The results were promising and surprisingly showed rapid clearance of lysososmal-storage vesicles in keratocytes and clearing of the cornea.

3.5. Corneal Wound Healing

Corneal wound healing plays an important role in the maintenance of corneal transparency and is thus crucial to normal visual function. Corneal scarring or opacity results from infection, physical trauma, excessive deposition of ECM, and/or angiogenesis. Corneal scarring is an important ocular pathology and is the third leading cause of blindness worldwide. Numerous growth factors and cytokines have been found to regulate corneal wound healing and include transforming growth factor beta (TGFβ), connective tissue growth factor, etc. Out of these cytokines TGFβ plays a central role in corneal wound healing, myofibroblast generation, and haze development. Studies also show that the opiod growth factor receptor pathway that decreases DNA synthesis also plays a critical role in regulating cell proliferation of the corneal epithelium leading to delayed wound healing. For the first time, Mohan et al. (2010), addressed AAV transgene delivery efficiency into keratocytes of normal and diseased (hazy and neovascularized) rabbit corneas *in vivo*. With different AAV serotypes we showed long term transgene expression of these vectors in the rabbit cornea after 4 months. Further work by our group also revealed that these vectors are suitable for corneal gene therapy, valuable in corneal wound healing, and also control corneal scarring as well as angiogenesis. Earlier we postulated that decorin gene delivery into rabbit and human keratocytes significantly reduced TGFβ-driven transdifferentiation of keratocytes to myofibroblasts *in vitro*. Recently we also tested AAV mediated decorin gene therapy and postulated that decorin gene therapy can be used to treat corneal haze *in vivo* (Mohan et al., 2010).

Acknowledgments

The work is supported by the RO1EY17294 (RRM) grant from the National Eye Institute, National Institutes of Health, Bethesda, Maryland, USA and a grant from the Research to Prevent Blindness, New York, New York, USA.

References

Bemelmans, A.P., Arsenijevic, Y., Majo F., (2009) Efficient lentiviral gene transfer into corneal stroma cells using a femtosecond laser. *Gene Therapy* 16: 933-938.

Bradshaw, J.J, Obritsch, W.F, Cho, B.J., Gregerson, D.S, Holland, E.J., (1999) *Ex vivo* transduction of corneal epithelial progenitor cells using a retroviral vector. *Investigative Ophthalmology & Visual Science* 40(1):230-235.

Collins, L., Fabre, J.W., (2004) A synthetic peptide vector system for optimal gene delivery to corneal endothelium. *The journal of gene medicine* 6:185–194.

de la Fuente, M., Seijo, B., Alonso, M.J., (2008) Novel hyaluronic acid-chitosan nanoparticles for ocular gene therapy. *Investigative Ophthalmology & Visual Science* 49: 2016–2024.

Hudde, T., Rayner, S.A., Comer, R.M, Weber, M., Isaacs, J.D., Waldmann, H., Larkin, D.F., George, A.J., (1999) Activated polyamidoamine dendrimers, a non-viral vector for gene transfer to the corneal endothelium. *Gene Therapy* 6 (5):939-943.

Hudde, T., Rayner, S.A., De, Alwis M., Thrasher, A.J., Smith, J., Coffin, R.S., George, A.J., Larkin, D.F., (2000) Adeno-associated and herpes simplex viruses as vectors for gene transfer to the corneal endothelium. *Cornea* 19(3):369-373.

Klebe, S., Sykes, P.J., Coster, D.J., Krishnan, R., Williams, K.A., (2001) Prolongation of sheep corneal allograft survival by *ex vivo* transfer of the gene encoding interleukin-10, *Transplantation* 71 (9):1214–1220.

Klebe, S., Stirling, J.W, Williams, K.A., (2000) Corneal endothelial cell nuclei are damaged after DNA transfer using a gene gun. *Clinical & Experimental Ophthalmology* 28(1):58-9.

Mohan, R.R., Gupta, R., Mehan, M.K., Cowden, J.W., Sinha, S., (2010) Decorin transfection suppresses profibrogenic genes and myofibroblast formation in human corneal fibroblasts. *Exp Eye Res.* 91(2):238-245.

Mohan, R.R., Schultz, G.S., Hong, J.W., Mohan, R.R., Wilson, S.E., (2003) Gene transfer into rabbit keratocytes using AAV and lipid-mediated plasmid DNA vectors with a lamellar flap for stromal access. *Exp Eye Res.* 76(3):373-383.

Mohan, R.R., Sharma, A., Netto, M.V., Sinha, S., Wilson, S.E., (2005) Gene therapy in the cornea. *Progress in Retinal and Eye Research* 24(5):537-559. Review.

Oral, H.B., Larkin, D.F., Fehervari, Z., Byrnes, A.P., Rankin, A.M., Haskard, D.O., Wood, M.J., Dallman, M.J., George, A.J., (1997) *Ex vivo* adenovirus-mediated gene transfer and immunomodulatory protein production in human cornea. *Gene Therapy* 4(7):639-647.

Oshima, Y., Sakamoto, T., Hisatomi, T., Tsutsumi, C., Sassa, Y., Ishibashi, T., Inomata, H., (2002) Targeted gene transfer to corneal stroma *in vivo* by electric pulses. *Exp Eye Res.* 74(2):191-198.

Oshima, Y., Sakamoto, T., Yamanaka, I., Nishi, T., Ishibashi, T., Inomata, H., (1998) Targeted gene transfer to corneal endothelium *in vivo* by electric pulse. *Gene Therapy* (10):1347-1354.

Parker, D.G,, Coster, D.J., Brereton, H.M., Hart, P.H., Koldej, R., Anson, D.S., Williams, K.A., (2010) Lentivirus-mediated gene transfer of interleukin 10 to the ovine and human cornea. *Clinical & Experimental Ophthalmology* 38(4):405-413.

Pleyer, U., Groth, D., Hinz, B., Keil, O., Bertelmann, E., Rieck, P., Reszka, R., (2001) Efficiency and toxicity of liposome-mediated gene transfer to corneal endothelial cells, *Exp Eye Res.* 73(1):1–7.

Qi, H., Shine, H.D., Li, D.Q., de, Paiva C.S., Farley, W.J., Jones, D.B., Pflugfelder, S.C., (2008) Glial cell-derived neurotrophic factor gene delivery enhances survival of human corneal epithelium in culture and the overexpression of GDNF in bioengineered constructs. *Exp Eye Res.* 87(6):580-586.

Saghizadeh, M., Kramerov, A.A., Yaghoobzadeh, Y., Hu, J., Ljubimova, J.Y., Black, K.L., Castro, M.G., Ljubimov, A.V., (2010) Adenovirus-driven overexpression of proteinases in organ-cultured normal human corneas leads to diabetic-like changes. *Brain Research Bulletin* 15:81(2-3):262-72.

Seitz, B., Baktanian, E., Gordon, E.M., Anderson, W.F., LaBree, L., McDonnell, P.J., (1998) Retroviral vector-mediated gene transfer into keratocytes: in vitro effects of polybrene and protamine sulfate. *Graefe's Arch Clin Exp Ophthalmol* 236(8):602-612.

Seitz, B., Moreira, L., Baktanian, E., Sanchez, D., Gray, B., Gordon, E.M., Anderson, W.F., McDonnell, P.J., Retroviral vector-mediated gene transfer into keratocytes in vitro and *in vivo*. *American Journal of Ophthalmology* 126(5):630-639.

Sharma, A., Tovey, J.C., Ghosh, A., Mohan, R.R., (2010) AAV serotype influences gene transfer in corneal stroma *in vivo*. *Exp Eye Res.* 91(3):440-448

Sharma, A., Ghosh, A., Siddappa, C., Mohan, R.R., (2010) Gene Therapy for the cornea, conjunctiva, and lacrimal gland. *Encyclopedia of the Eye.* Oxford: Academic Press; Edited by Darlene A. Dartt, Vol 2, 185-194.

Friedmann, T., and Roblin, R., (1972) Gene therapy for human genetic disease? *Science* 175:949Y955

Wang, I.J., Carlson, E.C., Liu, C.Y., Kao, C.W., Hu, F.R., Kao, W.W., (2002) Cis-regulatory elements of the mouse Krt1.12 gene. *Molecular Vision* 8:94-101.

Yamashita, T., Sonoda, S., Suzuki, R., Arimura, N., Tachibana, K., Maruyama, K., Sakamoto, T., (2007) A novel bubble liposome and ultrasound- mediated gene transfer to ocular surface: RC-1 cells in vitro and conjunctiva *in vivo*. *Exp Eye Res.* 85: 741–748.

Yang, J.G., Sun, N.X., Cui, L.J., Wang, X.H., Feng, Z.H., (2009) Adenovirus-mediated delivery of p27(KIP1) to prevent wound healing after experimental glaucoma filtration surgery. *Acta Pharmacologica· Sinica* 30(4):413-423.

In: Advances in Eye Research. Volume 1 ISBN 978-1-61324-169-1
Editor: William L. Thomsen, pp. 65-91

Chapter III

X- and Gamma Ray Interactions with Soft Contact Lenses

Murat Kurudirek**, Bekir Doğan and Neslihan Ekinci
Faculty of Science, Department of Physics, Ataturk University, 25240, Erzurum, Turkey

Abstract

In view of the extensive use of radioactive isotopes in medical fields such as nuclear diagnostics (computerized tomography), nuclear medicine, radiation dosimetry and radiation biophysics, the knowledge on X- and gamma ray interactions with different types of materials has become the subject of researches for nuclear engineers, radiologists and radiation physicists for different purposes i.e. shielding, dosimetry, X-ray imaging and radiotherapy. The photon mass attenuation and mass energy absorption coefficients, energy dependence, effective atomic number, effective electron density and buildup factor are the basic quantities required in determining the penetration of X- and gamma photons through the material. While the extensive studies based on radiation interaction in biological materials are available, there are almost no studies for soft contact lenses from the point of X- and gamma ray interactions. At this point, the present study aimed at the investigation of X and/or gamma

* Tel.: +90 442 2314167; fax: +90 442 2360948. e-mail address: mkurudirek@gmail.com

radiation interaction with different types of soft contact lenses in terms of the parameters viz. mass attenuation and energy absorption coefficients, effective atomic number, effective electron density and energy dependence in the wide energy range of 1 keV-20 MeV as well as the energy absorption and exposure buildup factors from 0.015 to 15 MeV up to 40 mfp penetration depth. The influences of photon energy, chemical composition and penetration depth on these parameters were studied.

Keywords: Soft contact lens, X and gamma rays, dosimetry, medical imaging, radiotherapy

Introduction

Millions of people all over the world face visionary problems. They need either glass spectacles or lenses to correct their visionary problems. The contact lenses are almost new in the medical sector compared to the eye glasses. But the popularity of the lenses is much more than that of the eye glasses. It has even been observed that many people have discarded their eye glasses and begun to use the lenses. Contact lenses are used as corrective, cosmetic, or therapeutic purpose. Corrective contact lenses are designed to improve vision. Conditions correctable with contact lenses include myopia, hypermetropia, astigmatism and presbyopia. Compared to spectacles, the contact lenses have major advantages. Contact lenses give a superior optical result, with a larger field of vision, no peripheral distortion, and no misting up in humid conditions. Furthermore, eye glasses are usually large and heavy. People often find these eye glasses pretty uncomfortable.

There have been many interesting historical inventions in the development of contact lenses. In 1930, the development of glass contact lenses provided some means of visual restoration, particularly for keratoconus patients. In 1947, plastic, polymethylmethacrylate (PMMA) corneal contact lenses were invented by Touhy. In 1952, Songes developed a smaller corneal lens. In 1960, Wichterle developed the hydromethylmethacryate (HEMA) soft contact lens. This was readily adopted by Bausch & Lomb and popularized in 1971. In 1974-1975, the cellulose acetate butryate (CAB) was developed. In 1975-1976, The Boston rigid gas permeable (RGP) lens was developed. By 1980, the development of the RGP contact lenses in the marketplace was expanded to the development of the small manufacturing laboratory.

Over the year, there has been continuing improvement in lenses and in their care systems that have made contact lenses comfortable for the individual patient. The concept of disposable lenses was first developed by Vistakon [1].

Contact lenses may be rigid or soft depending on the nature of the material composition. Extended-wear or prolonged –wear lenses are that are worn for 24 hours or more. Gas permeable lenses are lenses that permit the passage of oxygen and carbon dioxide. Although soft lenses do this, by convention the term gas permeable is used only for rigid lenses. The term rigid is primarily a departure from the word hard which was used fort he polymethylmethacrylate (PMMA) lenses. Cosmetic contact lenses are designed to change the appearance of the eye. People are willing to enhance their style and appearance. The majority of teenagers use the colored contact lenses. The colored lenses change the look of the person completely and make one look more attractive. A bandage lens is a contact lens that is used over the cornea to protect it from external influences and to permit healing underliying corneal disorders. Soft lenses may be also classified according to whether they are hydrophobic (fear water) or hydrophobic (love water). Soft lenses are made of two different materials, hydrogel and nonhydrogel. Most hydrogel soft lenses are made with hydroxyethylmethacrylate (HEMA) as their base ingredient but are often copolymerized with other materials. There are, however, other non-HEMA materials available such as glycerol methylmethacrylate.

Radiation interaction with matter became an important subject with the extensive use of gamma-active isotopes in various fields' viz. nuclear diagnostics (computerized tomography), radiation protection, nuclear medicine, radiation dosimetry, gamma ray fluorescence studies, radiation biophysics and etc. The absorbed dose is important in medical radiation therapy and dosimetry, whereas the attenuation of the incident beam is used in medical imaging [2]. While the photons in the keV range are important in radiation biology as well as in medical diagnostics and therapy, the photons in the MeV range are vital for radiography and medical imaging [3,4]. When a beam of X- and/or gamma rays falls on a layer of material, it is absorbed, scattered and/or transmitted by interaction of its photons with the atoms of this matter [5]. The photon mass attenuation and mass energy absorption coefficients, energy dependence, effective atomic number, effective electron density and buildup factor are the basic quantities required in determining the penetration of X- and gamma photons through the material. The mass attenuation coefficient (μ/ρ) is a measure of probability of interaction that occurs between incident photons and matter of unit mass per unit area [6]. The mass energy absorption coefficient (μ_{en}/ρ) which is a measure of the average fractional amount of incident photon energy transferred to kinetic energy of charged particles as a result of these interactions is of interest in estimating absorbed dose in medical and health physics and also in radiation shielding applications [7-9]. The μ_{en}/ρ is a basic physical quantity used in calculation of the energy deposition by X- and/or gamma rays in biological, shielding and other materials. The energy dependence (ED) is an important parameter because in order to select the most suitable detector for a given dose measurement, the dosimetric characteristics of the various materials must be known, in particular, their energy dependence [10]. The energy dependence of a given material can be defined as the ratio of the mass energy-absorption coefficient μ_{en}/ρ to that of air at a particular energy [11]. The effective atomic number and effective electron density are the basic and important quantities among the parameters determining the constitutive structure of an unknown object or material. Both of effective atomic number and effective electron density has physical meaning and gives basic information about the characteristics of a multi-element material. Using the constants like effective atomic number (Z_{eff}) and effective electron density (N_e) of multi-element materials, one can calculate the energy absorption in a given medium via well established formulas. Effective atomic number (Z_{eff}) is also such a useful parameter that in some cases viz. designing radiation shielding, computing absorbed dose and build-up factor, it represents radiation interaction with matter. In some cases, in order to have an initial information about the chemical composition of a material the Z_{eff} can be utilized. For example the materials having large Z_{eff} generally corresponds to the inorganic compounds and metals, while a small Z_{eff} (≤ 10) is an indicator of organic substances [3]. The effective atomic numbers are useful in medical radiation dosimetry for the calculation of dose in radiation therapy and medical imaging, where the cross-sectional anatomy is generated by computer-assisted tomography (CAT) scans [12]. In composite materials like soft contact lenses, it is quite reasonable to define an effective atomic number, Z_{eff} to describe the properties of an alloy in terms of an equivalent element. Effective atomic number of a multi-element material which is a very useful parameter for many fields of scientific applications is similar to that atomic number of elements. However, on the basis of Hine's expression [13] that the effective atomic number of a material composed of several elements can not be expressed by a single number, it can be concluded that it is an energy dependent parameter due to the dominance of different partial photon interaction processes in different energy regions. In the medical and biological context, gamma ray buildup factor is of importance in distribution of photon flux and in calculation of radiation dose received by the biological materials in addition to the importance of knowledge on other photon interaction parameters such as mass attenuation coefficients and effective atomic numbers [14]. In some cases, while shield designing or estimating the absorbed dose, the secondary radiation can occur due to buildup of photons which arise from the collided part of the incident beam. When photons enter the medium/body, they degrade their energy and buildup in the medium, giving rise to secondary radiation which can be estimated by the 'buildup factor' [15]. There are two types of buildup factor: a) the energy absorption buildup factor that is the buildup factor in which the quantity of interest is the absorbed or deposited energy in the interacting material and the detector response function is that of absorption in the interacting material, b) the exposure buildup factor is the buildup factor in which the quantity of interest is the exposure and the detector response function is that of absorption in air [16]. There are different available methods to calculate the buildup factor such as G-P fitting method [17] and invariant embedding method [18-20]. Recently, American National Standards ANSI/ANS 6.4.3 [21] has provided buildup factor data for 23 elements, one compound and two mixtures (i.e. air and water) and concrete at energies in the range 0.015-15 MeV up to penetration depths of 40 mean free path by using the G-P method. The developed G-P fitting formula is known to be accurate within a few percent error [17,22]. Recently, Harima has made an extensive historical review and an assessment for the status of buildup factor calculations and applications [23].

At this point, the present study aimed at the investigation of X and/or gamma radiation interaction with different types of soft contact lenses in terms of the parameters mass attenuation and energy absorption coefficients, effective atomic number, effective electron density and energy dependence in the wide energy range of 1keV-20MeV as well as the energy absorption and exposure buildup factors from 0.015 to 15 MeV up to 40 mfp penetration depths. The influences of photon energy, chemical composition and penetration depth on these parameters were studied.

Theory

Total Mass Attenuation and Mass Energy Absorption Coefficient

According to the Lambert-Beer law, a parallel beam of monoenergetic X-ray and γ- ray photons is attenuated in matter by the following exponential attenuation equation

$$I = I_0 e^{(-\frac{\mu}{\rho})t}, \quad (1)$$

where I_0 and I are the incident intensity of photons without attenuation and the attenuated intensity of photons in the sample, respectively, $t(g/cm^2)$ is the areal density of the sample, $\mu/\rho(cm^2/g)$ is the total mass attenuation coefficient $(TMAC)$ which is a density independent quantity.

In case of a multi-element material (i.e. chemical compound or homogeneous mixture) constituting the sample, the mass attenuation coefficient can be obtained from the coefficients for the constituent elements according to the weighted average

$$\mu/\rho = \sum_i W_i (\mu/\rho)_i \quad (2)$$

where W_i is the proportion by weight of the i th constituent element.

The mass energy absorption coefficients $(MEAC)$ of the given materials can be obtained from Eq. (2) by substituting the mass energy absorption coefficient for the mass attenuation coefficient. However, it should be mentioned that the Eq. (2) is valid for mass energy absorption under the assumption that the errors in calculating mass energy absorption coefficients are small for photon energies below 20 MeV [8].

Effective Atomic Number, Electron Density and Energy Dependence

The effective atomic numbers of the soft contact lenses have been obtained by means of the practical formula [24]:

$$Z_{PI\,eff} = \frac{\sum_i f_i A_i (\frac{\mu}{\rho})_i}{\sum_j f_j \frac{A_j}{Z_j} (\frac{\mu}{\rho})_j} \tag{3}$$

where f_i is the fraction by mole of the each constituent element providing that $\sum_i f_i = 1$, A_i is the atomic weight, Z_j is the atomic number, $(\frac{\mu}{\rho})_i$ is the mass attenuation coefficient. The effective atomic number for photon energy absorption ($Z_{PEA_{eff}}$) can be obtained from Eq. (3) by substituting the mass energy absorption coefficient for the mass attenuation coefficient.

Also, the effective electron density is expressed by the following relation [24]:

$$N_E = N_A \frac{nZ_{eff}}{\sum_i n_i A_i} = N_A \frac{Z_{eff}}{\langle A \rangle} (electrons/g) \tag{4}$$

where $\langle A \rangle$ is the average atomic mass of the material. Thus, using the obtained values of Z_{eff} one can calculate the values of N_E by using the Eq. (4).

The kinetic energy released per unit mass (kerma) is defined as the initial kinetic energy of all secondary charged particles liberated per unit mass at a point of interested by uncharged radiation [7,11]. To obtain the relationship between kerma and mass energy absorption coefficient, let ψ (Jm^{-2}) be the energy fluence of mono-energetic photons passing normally through an area A in an absorber. Keeping in mind the energy transferred to charged particles and the mass in the volume with density ρ being $\psi A\mu_{en}dx$ and ρAdx, respectively, the kerma is then [25]

$$K = \frac{\psi A\mu_{en}dx}{\rho Adx} = \psi(\frac{\mu_{en}}{\rho}). \tag{6}$$

Since the kerma is the product of the energy fluence and the mass energy absorption coefficient, kerma of a material relative to air also known as the energy dependence can be expressed as the ratio between the mass energy absorption coefficient of the used material and the mass energy absorption coefficient of air [7]:

$$ED = \frac{(\mu_{en}/\rho)_{Material}}{(\mu_{en}/\rho)_{Air}} \tag{7}$$

Energy Absorption and Exposure Buildup Factors

To calculate the buildup factors, the G-P fitting parameters were obtained by the method of interpolation from the equivalent atomic number (Z_{eq}). Computations are illustrated step by step as follows:

a) Calculation of the equivalent atomic number, Z_{eq}
b) Calculation of geometric progression (G-P) fitting parameters
c) Calculation of energy absorption and exposure buildup factors

At the first step, the equivalent atomic number, Z_{eq} for a particular material has been calculated by matching the ratio, $(\mu/\rho)_{Compton}/(\mu/\rho)_{Total}$ of that material at a specific energy with the corresponding ratio of an element at the same energy. Thus, firstly the Compton partial mass attenuation coefficient, $(\mu/\rho)_{Compton}$, and the total mass attenuation coefficients, $(\mu/\rho)_{Total}$ were obtained for the elements of $Z = 4-40$ and for the chosen materials in the energy region 0.015-15 MeV, using the WinXCom computer program [26,27] (initially developed as XCOM [28]). For the interpolation of

Z_{eq} for which the ratio $(\mu/\rho)_{Compton}/(\mu/\rho)_{Total}$ lies between two successive ratios of elements, the following formula has been employed:

$$Z_{eq} = \frac{Z_1(\log R_2 - \log R) + Z_2(\log R - \log R_1)}{\log R_2 - \log R_1} \tag{8}$$

where Z_1 and Z_2 are the atomic numbers of elements corresponding to the ratios R_1 and R_2 respectively, R is the ratio for the chosen building materials at a specific energy.

At the second step, to calculate the G-P fitting parameters a similar interpolation procedure was adopted as in the case of the equivalent atomic number. The G-P fitting parameters for elements were taken from the ANSI/ANS-6.4.3 [21] standard reference database which provides the G-P fitting parameters for elements from beryllium to iron in the energy region 0.015-15 MeV up to 40 mfp.

At the final step, these parameters were used to calculate the energy absorption and exposure buildup factors from the G-P fitting formula [18]:

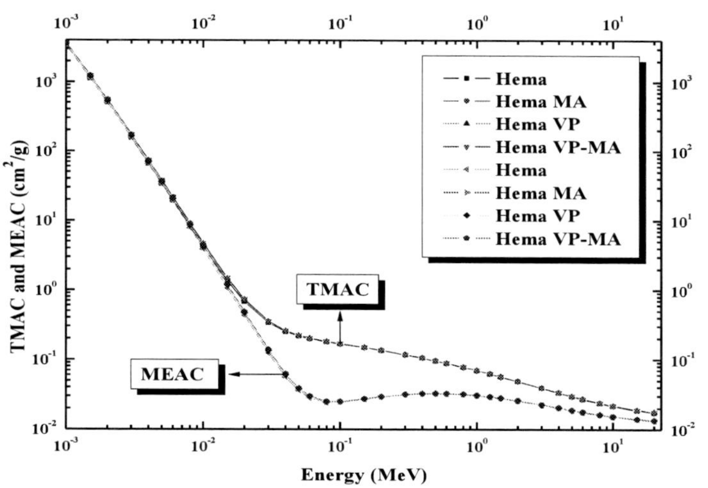

Figure 1. Total mass attenuation $(TMAC)$ and mass energy absorption $(MEAC)$ coefficients of the given materials for total photon interaction from 1 keV to 100 GeV.

$$B(E,X) = 1 + \frac{b-1}{K-1}(K^x - 1) \text{ for } K \neq 1 \tag{9}$$

$$B(E,X) = 1 + (b-1)x \text{ for } K = 1 \tag{10}$$

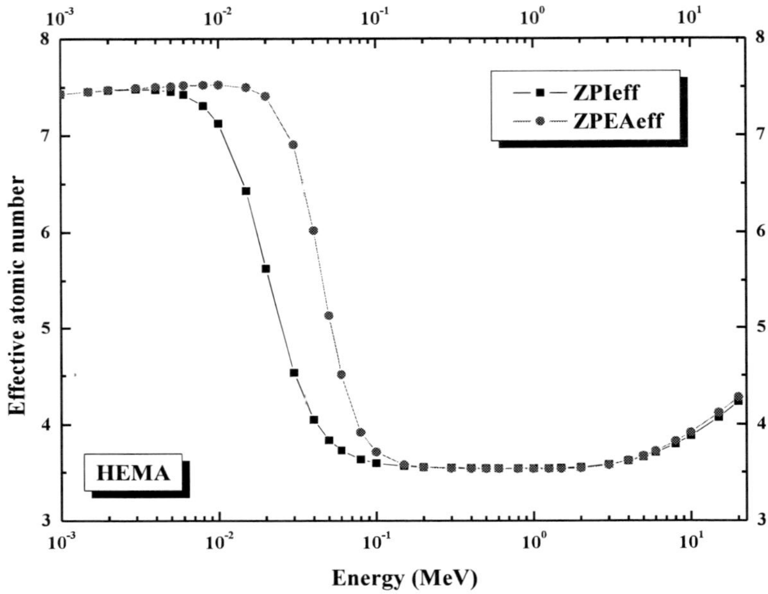

a)

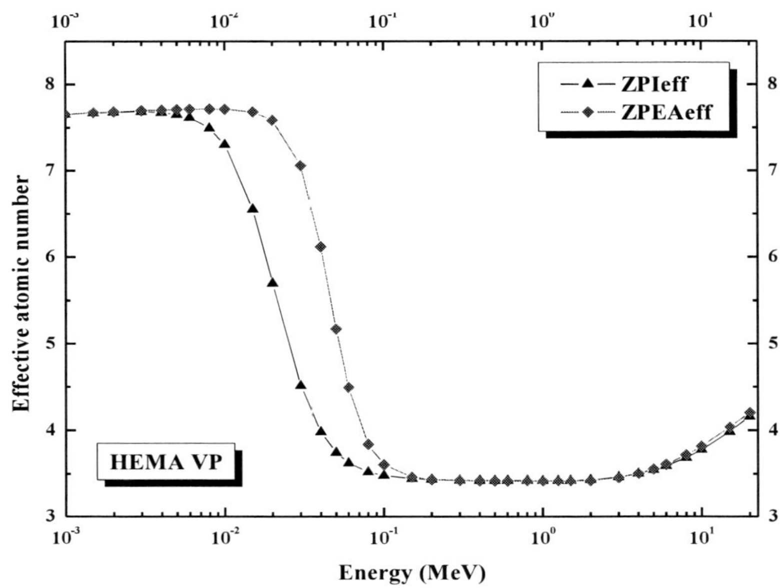

b)

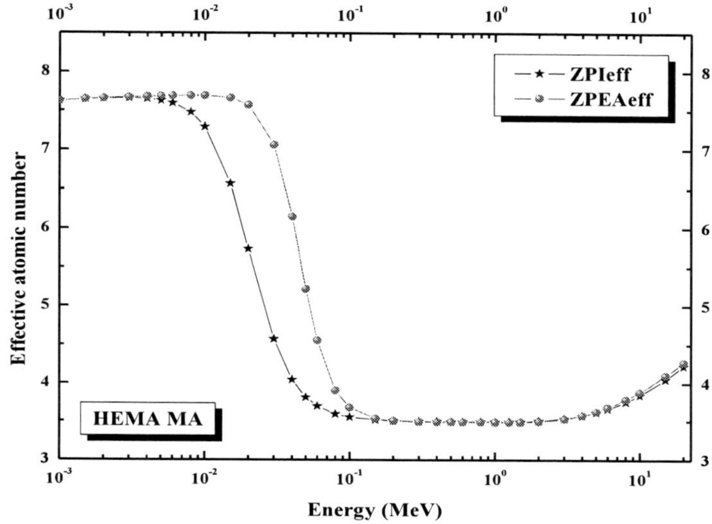

c)

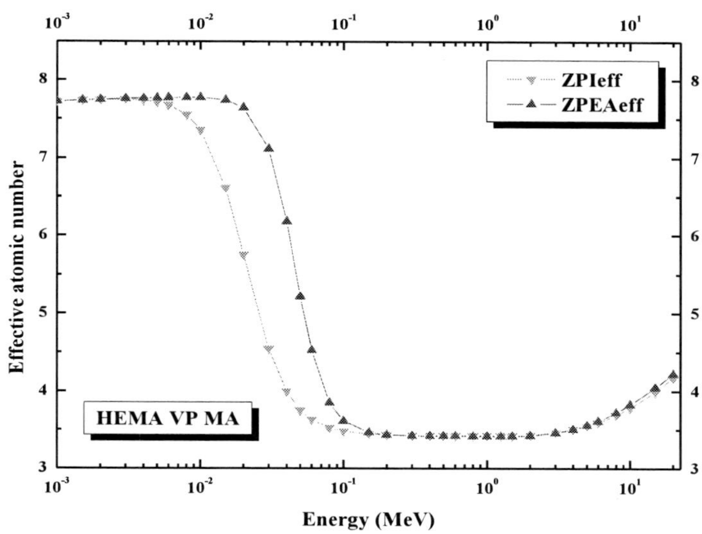

d)

Figure 2. (a,b,c,d) Effective atomic numbers of the given materials from 1 keV to 20 MeV.

where,

$$K(E,x) = cx^{a} + d\frac{\tanh(x/X_k - 2) - \tanh(-2)}{1 - \tanh(-2)} \quad \text{for } x \leq 40mfp \quad (11)$$

where E is the incident photon energy, x is the penetration depth in mfp, a,b,c,d and X_k are the G-P fitting parameters and b is the value of buildup factor at 1 mfp. The parameter K represents the photon dose multiplication and the change in the shape of the spectrum.

Calculations

Mass attenuation coefficients of soft contact lenses and elements constituting the soft contact lenses have been calculated by the WinXCom program. This program provides total cross-sections and attenuation coefficients of elements, compounds or mixtures as well as partial cross-sections for incoherent and coherent scattering, photoelectric absorption and pair production both in the field of nucleus and electrons at energies from 1 keV to 100 GeV [26,27].

Results

Total Mass Attenuation and Mass Energy Absorption Coefficients, Effective Atomic Number and Electron Density

The total mass attenuation and mass energy absorption coefficients of soft contact lenses have been shown in Fig. 1. It has been observed that both of $TMAC$ and $MEAC$ decrease with the increase in energy. At the intermediate energy region where Compton scattering is the main photon interaction process, the $MEAC$ has lower values than $TMAC$ due to the state that Compton scattering is of less importance for $MEAC$ than $TMAC$. For the given materials the effective atomic numbers, Z_{eff} have been calculated using Eq. (4). In the present work, the mass attenuation coefficients of soft contact lenses have been calculated using WinXCom [26,27]. The values of the effective electron density, N_e, have been calculated by the use of Eq. (5). From the Figure 2 (a,b,c,d) it can be concluded that the effective atomic numbers of soft contact lenses vary with photon energy. The variations of the effective atomic numbers in different energy regions depend on the mainly three photon interaction processes namely the photoelectric absorption, Compton scattering and the pair production. The maximum and minimum values of effective atomic numbers for soft contact lenses have been found in the low energy region (<100 keV for photon interaction and <200 keV for photon energy absorption) and in intermediate energy region where photoelectric absorption and Compton scattering are dominating, respectively (Figure 2 (a,b,c,d)). The all variations can be clearly explained by the Z dependence of total atomic cross sections thus effective atomic numbers as Z^{4-5} for photoelectric absorption, Z for Compton scattering and Z^2 for pair production.

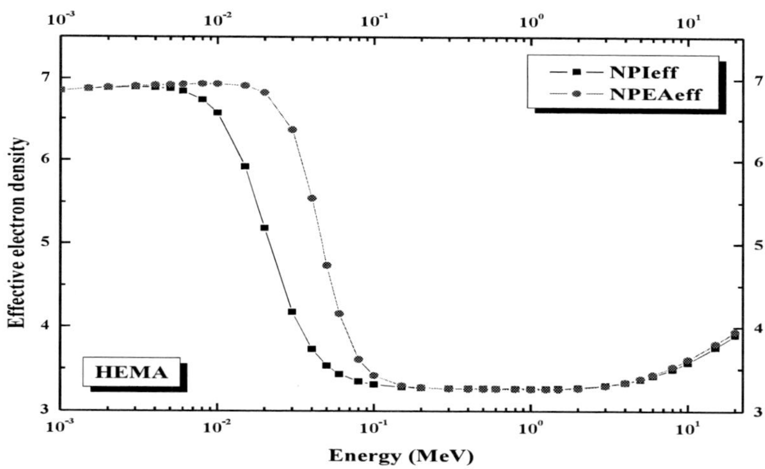

a)

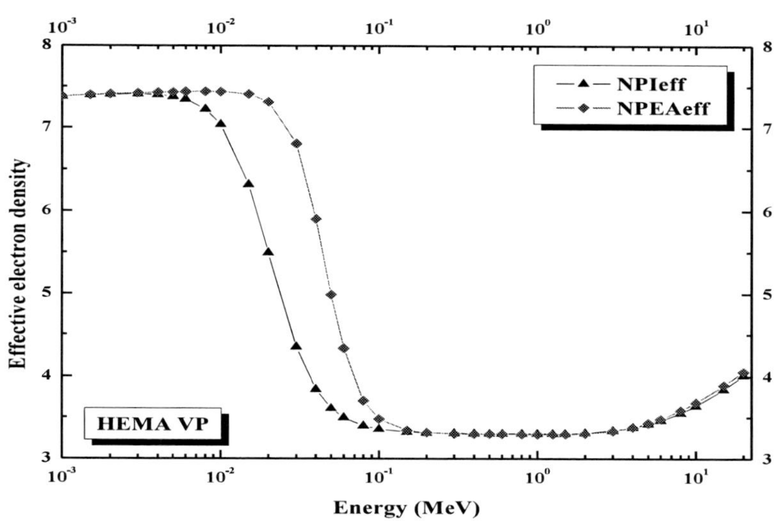

b)

Figure 3. (Continued)

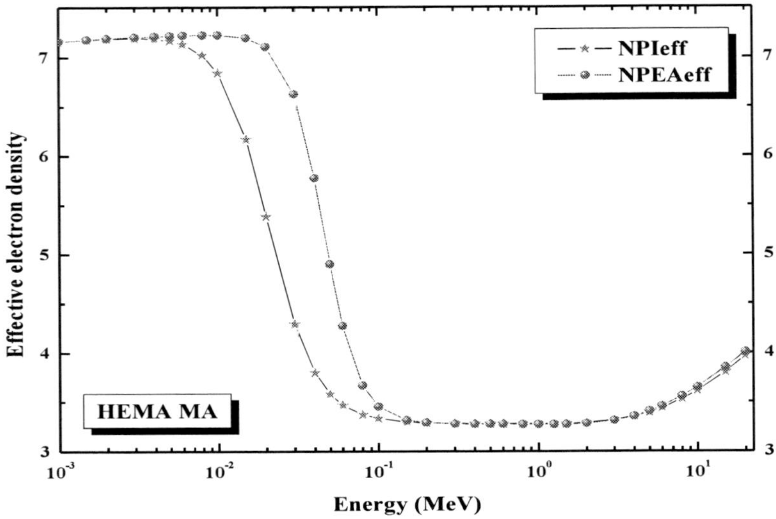

c)

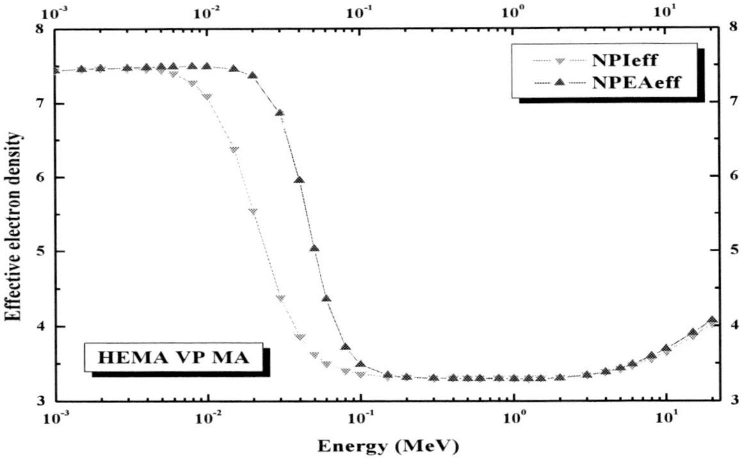

d)

Figure 3. (a,b,c,d) Effective electron densities of the given materials from 1 keV to 20 MeV.

The variation of effective electron densities (N_e) with incident photon energy is shown in Figure 3 (a,b,c,d). The decreasing trends observed are almost similar to the trends observed for effective atomic numbers. Therefore, the energy dependence of effective electron density shows the similar behavior based on partial photon interaction processes with matter. In contrast, no well chemical composition dependence of effective electron density has been observed in the present study.

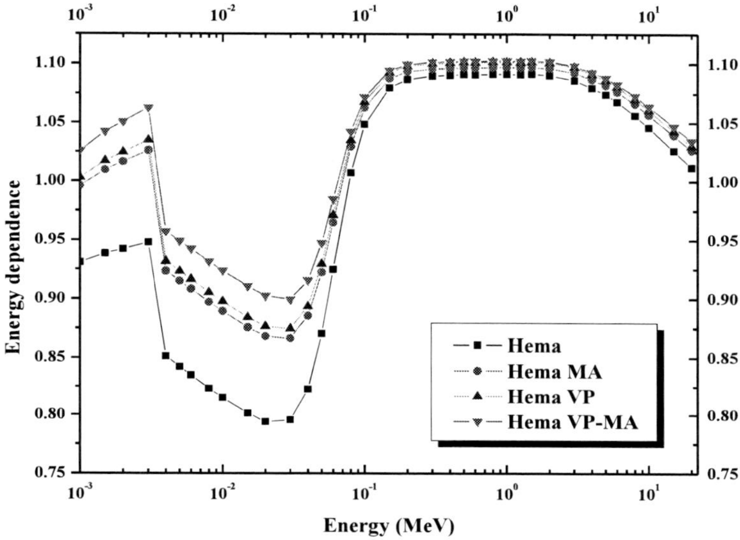

Figure 4. Energy dependences (ED) of the given materials from 1 keV to 20 MeV.

Energy Dependence

The variation of energy dependence (ED) with energy is shown in Fig. 4. On the basis of the relative domination of the partial photon interaction processes, viz., photoelectric absorption, Compton scattering and pair production, it is worth mentioning that the variation of ED with energy is clear. The values of ED for the soft contact lenses have maximum values in the intermediate energy region where Compton scattering is the main interaction process whereas the minimum values observed in the low energy region where photoelectric absorption is the main interaction process.

Table 1. Chemical concentrations of soft contact lenses

Concentration of Soft Contact Lenses (%)			
Soft Contact Lenses			H_2O
Hema	$(C_6H_{10}O_3)$	62	38
Hema-MA	$(C_{10}H_{16}O_5)$	42	58
Hema-VP	$(C_{12}H_{19}NO_4)$	34	66
Hema-VP MA	$(C_{16}H_{25}NO_6)$	29	71

EABF and *EBF*

The gamma ray buildup, which represents the collided part of the incident gamma rays, mainly arises from the larger penetration depths (especially for materials of larger thickness) and divergence of the incident beam. It can be clearly seen from the figures that the values of *EABF* and *EBF* are always larger than unity.

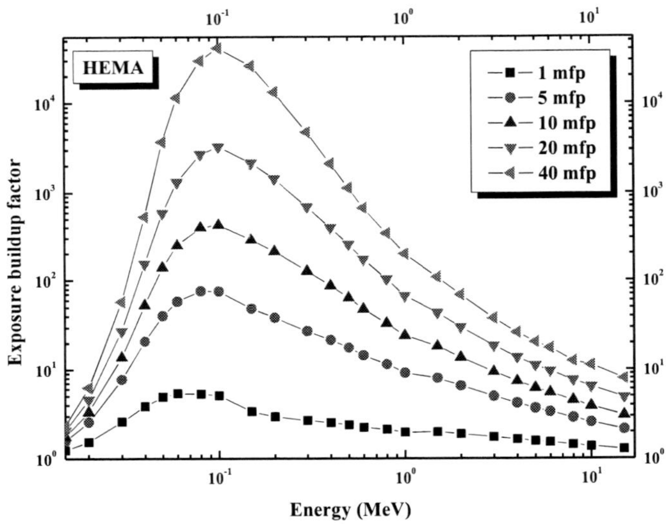

a)

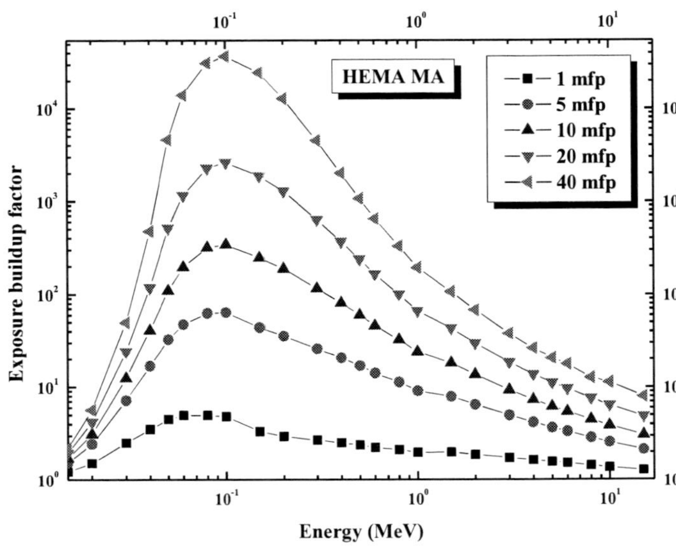

b)

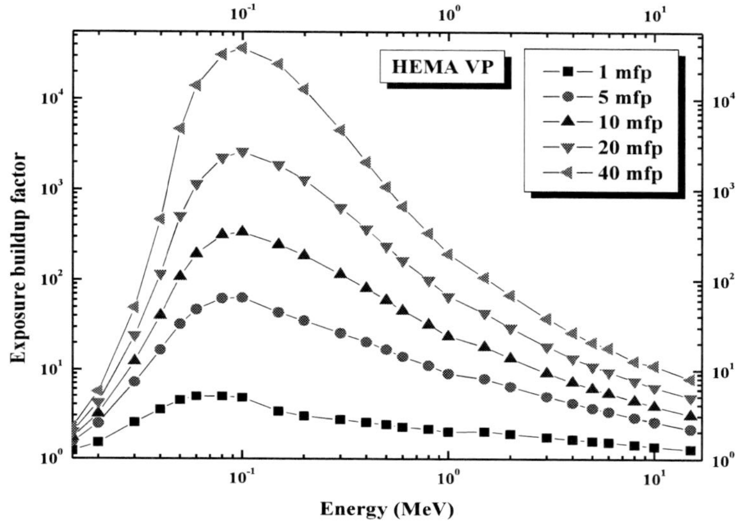

c)

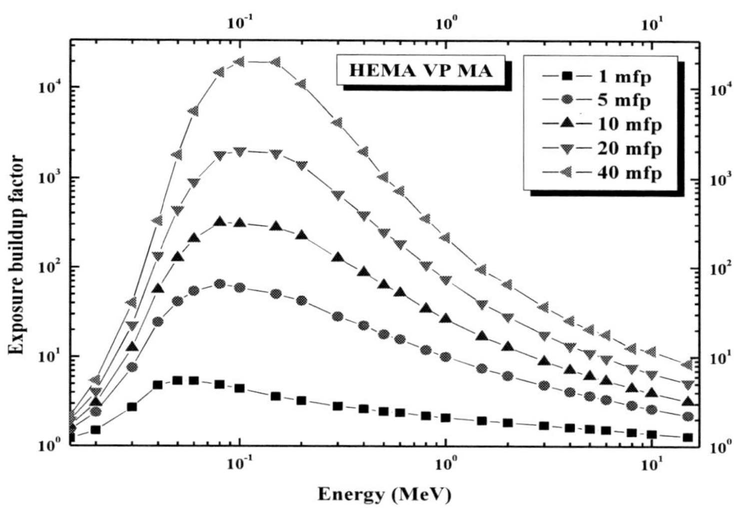

d)

Figure 6. (a,b,c,d,e) The exposure buildup factor in the energy region 0.015-15 MeV at 1,5,10,20,40 mfp.

Figures 5,6 (a,b,c,d) show $EABF$ and EBF at fixed penetration depths from 0.015 to 15 MeV. It is seen that initially, the $EABF$ and EBF values start increasing with the increase in photon energy up to a maximum value at intermediate energies, then starts decreasing further with the increase in energy. This state can be clearly explained by the domination of different photon interaction processes at different energy regions. The absorption processes, namely photoelectric absorption and pair production lead to completely removal of photons, thus less buildup occurs at lower and high energy regions, whereas in the case of the scattering processes i.e. Compton scattering, the photons are not completely removed but their energies are only degraded. Hence, this process results with more multiple scattered photons which lead to increase in buildup of photons in the medium.

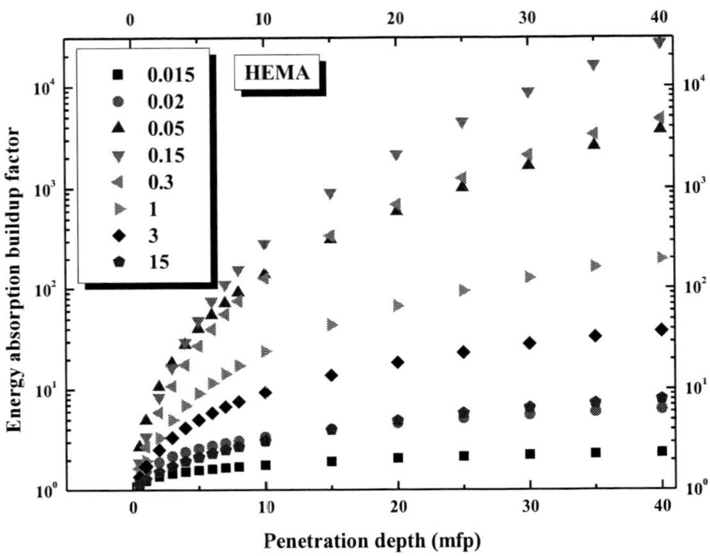

a)

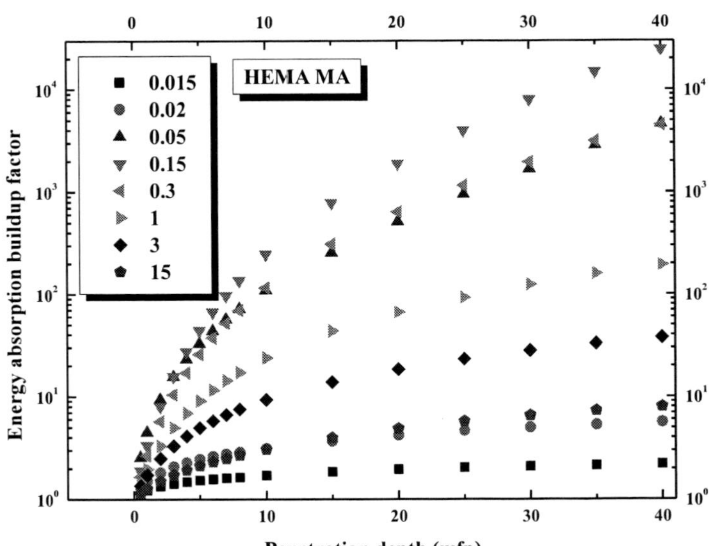

b)

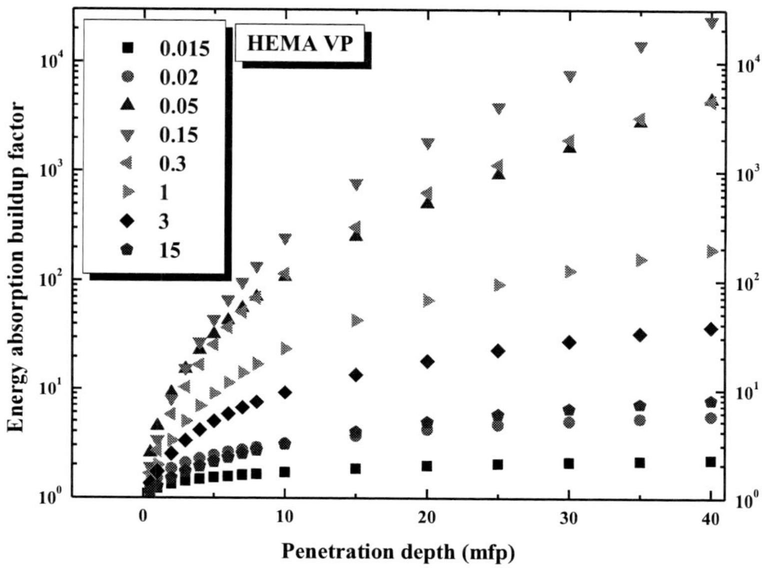

c)

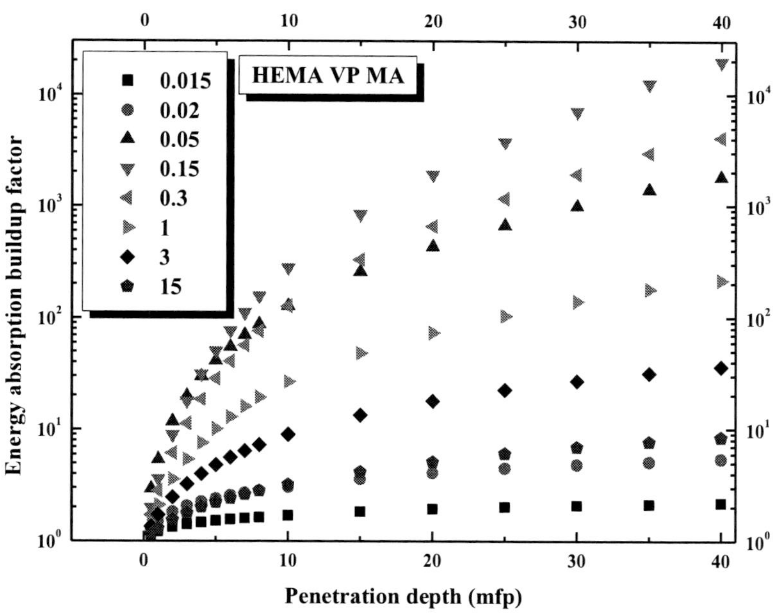

d)

Figure 7. (a,b,c,d) The energy absorption buildup factor up to 40 mfp at 0.015, 0.02, 0.05, 0.15, 0.3, 1, 3, 15 MeV.

The values of $EABF$ and EBF have been shown as a function of penetration depth in Figures 7,8 (a,b,c,d). It has been shown that with the increasing penetration depths; the $EABF$ and EBF also increase for the given materials due to the increase in number of scattered photons.

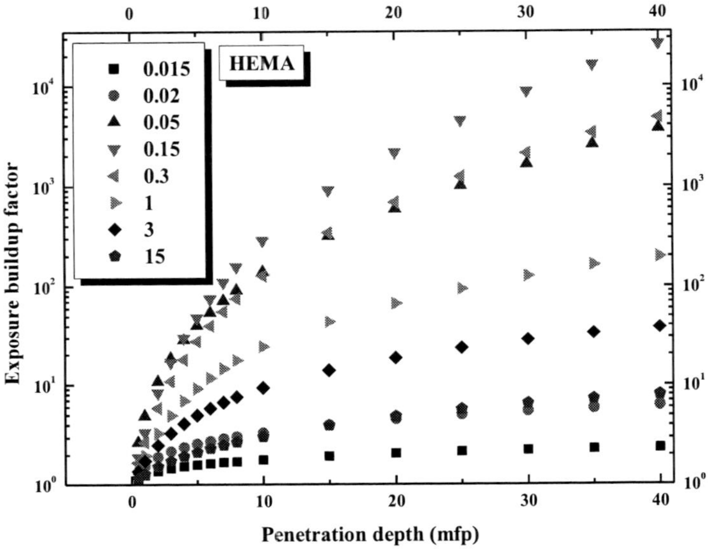

a)

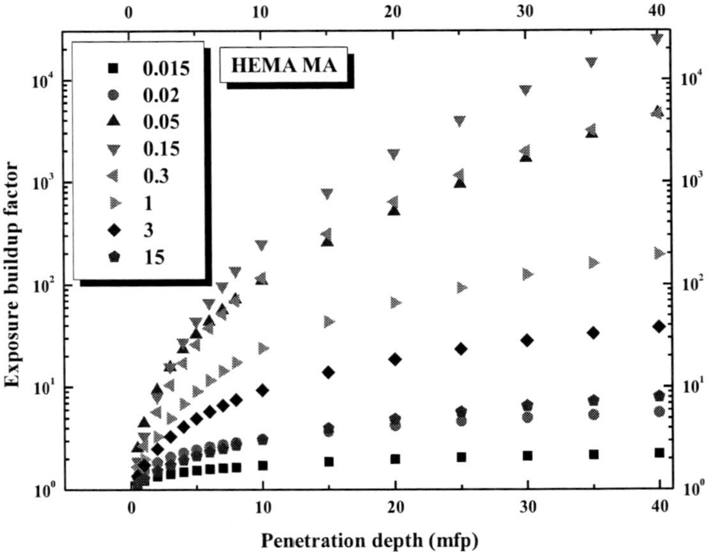

b)

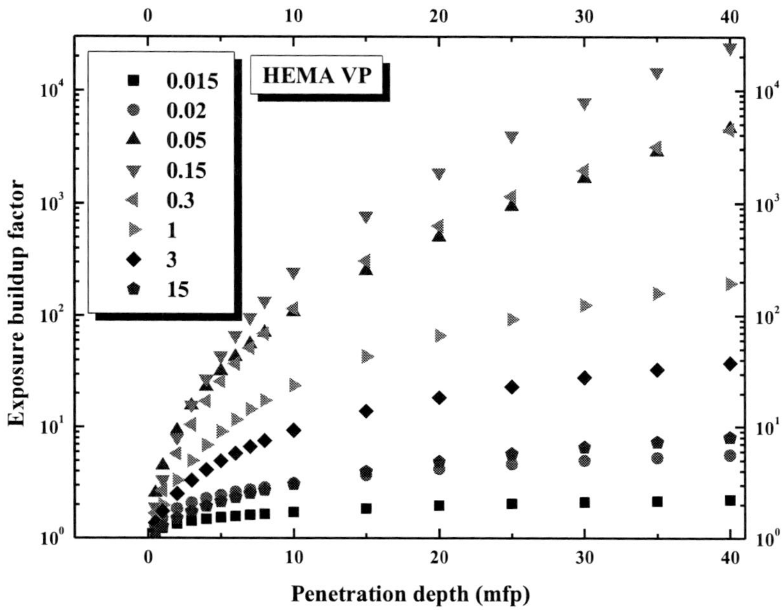

c)

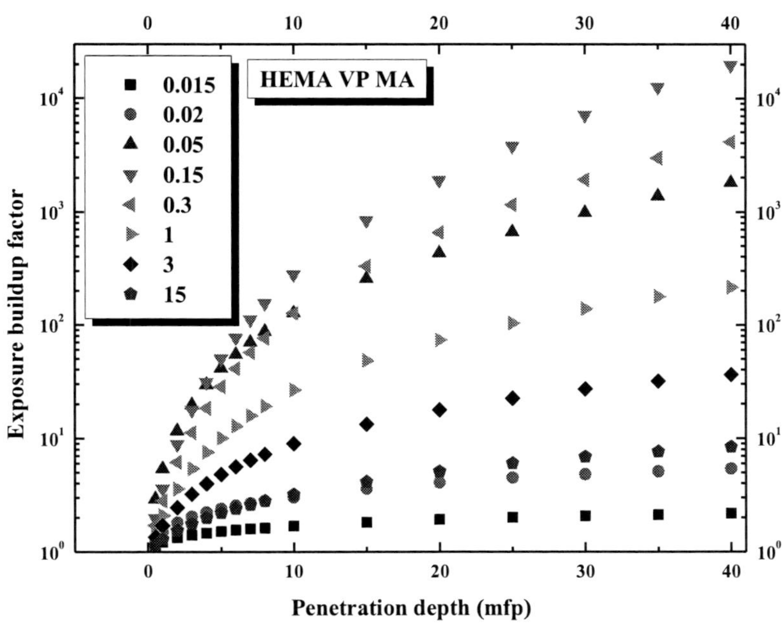

d)

Figure 8. (a,b,c,d) The exposure buildup factor up to 40 mfp at 0.015, 0.02, 0.05, 0.15, 0.3, 1, 3, 15 MeV.

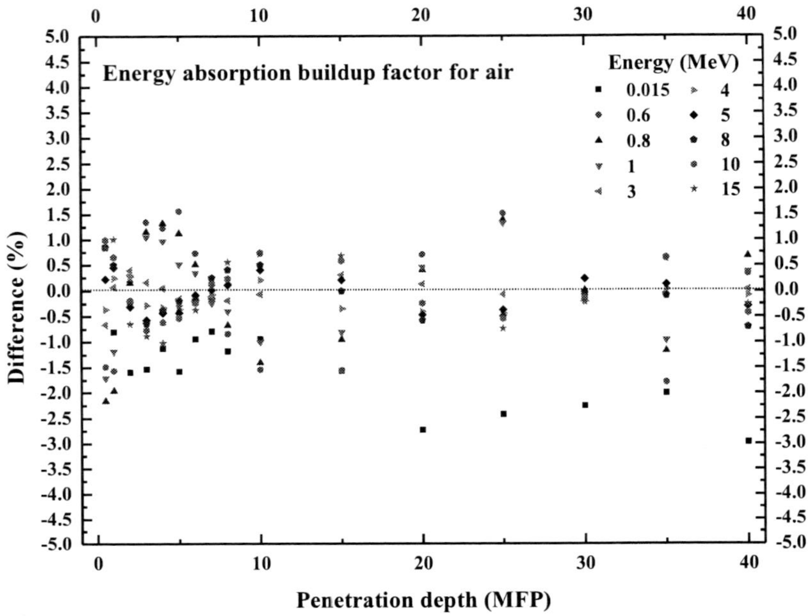

a)

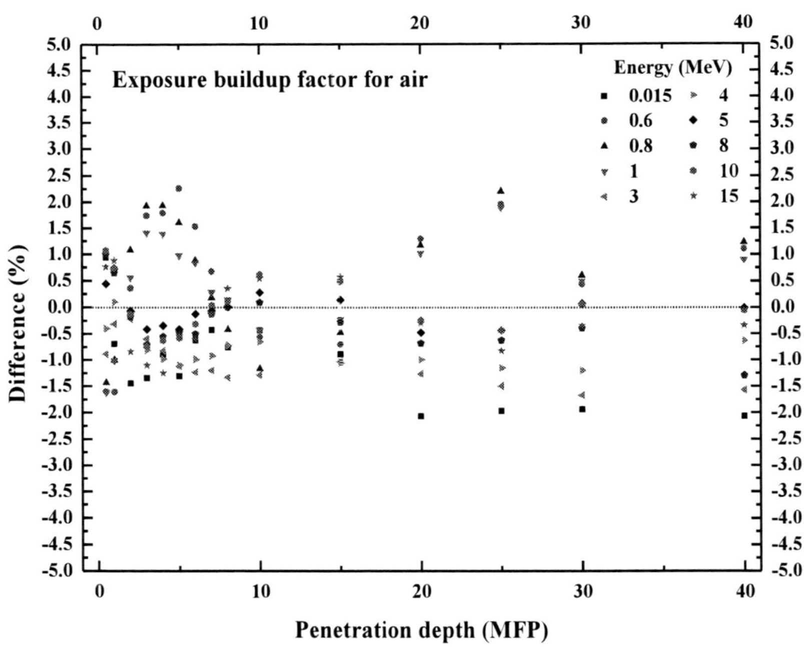

b)

Figure 9. (a,b) Difference (%) between ANSI database and present work with respect to the calculated values of $EABF$ and EBF for air at some energies up to 40 mfp.

Calculation Uncertainty

The accuracy of the calculated values of parameters related with photon interaction and energy absorption is based on mass attenuation coefficients. The mass attenuation coefficients of the elements have been taken from the WinXCom [26,27] database which is the successor of the XCom [28] database. WinXCom is a very useful computer program that one can calculate the mass attenuation coefficients of elements, compounds and mixtures for total and partial photon interaction processes with its facilitating to export the cross sectional data to a predefined MS Excel template which is further used for graphical or numerical progresses. Recently, it was reported by Hubbell [4] that the envelope of the uncertainty of mass attenuation coefficient is of the order of 1-2% in the energy range from 5 keV to a few MeV. In case of the energies of 1 to 4 keV, the discrepancies are known to reach to a value of 25 to 50%. Recently, Chantler has successfully addressed the huge discrepancies below 4 keV and derived new theoretical results of substantially higher accuracy in near-edge soft X-ray regions in detail [29]. The most interested energies widely used in biological, medical and shielding applications cover the energies larger than 5 keV, hence the presented results for building materials have an uncertainty of a few percentages. With respect to the accuracy of the calculated values of $EABF$ and EBF, it should be noted that calculations have been checked by comparing $EABF$ and EBF for air present in ANSI [21] database with our calculated $EABF$ and EBF for air in the energy region 0.015-15 MeV and penetration depth up to 40 mfp. From the Figure 9 it can be clearly seen that our calculated values for air agree well with that of ANSI [21] database within a few percent uncertainty. Recently, Asano and Sakamoto have evaluated the buildup factors of two typical heavy concretes to improve the capability of the various materials for the shielding wall by using the Monte Carlo simulation code, EGS4 [30]. They also compared their calculated values by that of concrete in ANSI/ANS-6.4.3 [21] standard reference database. Both of the calculations are in good agreement except for the slight differences which may be due to a) the ANSI/ANS data are based on the calculation result data by using the moments method [31] with parallel beam source and the Monte Carlo code, EGS4 with isotropic emission source, b) the development of the low energy photon treatments in EGS4 such as K-X ray, L-X ray and Bremsstrahlung. It was shown by Shimizu et al. [20] that the methods based on invariant embedding, G.P fitting and

Monte Carlo simulation agree well for 18 low-Z materials within small discrepancies. In the present study, the used soft contact lenses extremely consist of low Z elements i.e. H, C, N and O. Chemical concentrations of these elements have been presented Table 1. Hence, the used materials can be considered as low Z_{eq} materials. When compared with other available approximations such as Berger, Taylor and three exponential, the geometric-progression (G.P) fitting seem to reproduce the buildup factors with better accuracy. Harima et al. [17] have shown that the absolute values of maximum deviations of exposure build factors for water in G. P. fitting is within 0.5-3%, in three-exponential approach is within 0.4-9.3%, in Berger approach is within 0.9-42.7% and in Taylor approximation is within 0.4-53.2%.

Conclusion

Although the different types of radiation are not only hazardous for living organisms but also hazardous for other materials i.e. laboratory equipments, on the other hand the X- and gamma rays have been widely used for therapeutic purposes in medical fields such as nuclear diagnostics (computerized tomography), nuclear medicine, radiation dosimetry and radiation biophysics. The absorbed dose is important in medical radiation therapy and dosimetry, whereas the attenuation of the incident beam is used in medical imaging [2]. While the photons in the keV range are important in radiation biology as well as in medical diagnostics and therapy, the photons in the MeV range are vital for radiography and medical imaging [3,4]. Thus, the knowledge of photon interaction parameters such as photon mass attenuation and mass energy absorption coefficients, energy dependence, effective atomic number, effective electron density and buildup factor is of importance. Accurate values of these parameters are needed to provide essential data in diverse fields mentioned above. This work reports data on photon interaction parameters in the continuous energy region for some soft contact lenses namely hema, hema ma, hema vp and hema vp ma. The X- and gamma ray interactions with this type of materials have been presented and discussed in the present study.

References

[1] Stein, A.H.; Harrison, K.; Contact lenses after refractive surgery. *Ophthalmology Clinics of North America.* 9, 77.

[2] Manohara, S. R.; Hanagodimath, S. M.; Gerward, L. The effective atomic numbers of some biomolecules calculated by two methods: A comparative study. *Med. Phys.* 2009, 36, 137-141.

[3] Manohara, S. R., Hanagodimath, S. M., Gerward, L., 2008. Studies on effective atomic number, electron density and kerma for some fatty acids and carbohydrates. *Phys. Med. Biol.* 53, 377-386.

[4] Hubbell, J. H. Review of photon interaction cross section data in the medical and biological context. *Physics in Medicine and Biology* 1999, 44, R1-R22.

[5] El-Kateb, A. H., Rizk, R. A. M., Abdul-Kader, A. M., 2000. Determination of atomic cross-sections and effective atomic numbers for some alloys. *Annals of Nuclear Energy* 27, 1333-1343.

[6] Manohara, S. R.; Hanagodimath, S. M. Studies on effective atomic numbers and electron densities of essential aminoacids in the energy range 1 keV-100 GeV. *Nucl. Instr. And Meth.* B 2007, 258, 321-328.

[7] Manohara, S. R.; Hanagodimath, S. M. Effective atomic numbers for photon energy absorption of essential amino acids in the energy range 1 keV to 20 MeV. *Nucl. Instr. And Meth.* B 2007, 264, 9-14.

[8] Hubbell, J.H.; Seltzer, S.M.; 1995. Tables of X- ray mass attenuation coefficients and mass energy absorption coefficients from 1 keV to 20 MeV for elements Z=1 to 92 and 48 additional substances of dosimetric interest National Institute of Standards and Technology Gaithersburg, MD20899, Report NISTIR 5632.

[9] Manohara, S. R., Hanagodimath, S. M., Gerward, L., 2009. Photon interaction and energy absorption in glass: A transparent gamma ray shield. *Journal of Nuclear Materials* 393, 465-472.

[10] Shivaramu, V., Ramprasath 2000. Effective atomic numbers for photon energy absorption and energy dependence of some thermoluminescent dosimetric compounds *Nucl. Instr. And Meth.* B 168, 294-304.

[11] Attix, F. H. *Introduction to Radiological Physics and Radiation Dosimetry* (New York: Wiley) 1986.

[12] Jackson, D.F., Hawkes, D. J. X-ray attenuation coefficients of elements and mixtures. *Phys. Reports* 70 (1981) 169.

[13] Hine, G. J. 1952. The effective atomic numbers of materials for various gamma interactions. *Phys. Rev*. 85, 725.

[14] B. Chilton, J. K. Shultis, R. Faw, 1984. *Principle of Radiation Shielding*. Prentice Hall, Englewood Cliffs, New Jersey.

[15] Sidhu G S, Singh S P, Mudahar S G 2000 A study of energy and effective atomic number dependence of the exposure buildup factors in biological samples *Journal of Radiological Protection* 20 53-68.

[16] Singh, S. P., Singh, T., Kaur, P. 2008 Variation of energy absorption buildup factors with incident photon energy and penetration depth for some commonly used solvents Ann. *Nucl. Energy* 35, 1093-1097.

[17] Harima, Y., Sakamoto, Y., Tanaka, S., Kawai, M. 1986 Validity of the geometric-progression formula in approximating gamma ray build up factors *Nucl. Sci. Eng*. 94, 24-35.

[18] Sakamoto, Y., Tanaka, S. 1988 Interpolation of gamma ray buildup factors for point isotropic source with respect to atomic number *Nucl. Sci. Eng*. 100, 33-42.

[19] Shimizu, A 2002 Calculations of gamma-ray buildup factors up to depths of 100 mfp by the method of invariant embedding, (I) analysis of accuracy and comparison with other *data J. Nucl. Sci. Technol. 39*, 477.

[20] Shimizu, A., Onda, T., Sakamoto, Y. 2004 Calculations of gamma-ray buildup factors up to depths of 100 mfp by the method of invariant embedding, (III) generation of an improved data *set Nucl. Sci. Technol.* 41, 413-424.

[21] ANSI/ANS-6.4.3. 1991 Gamma ray attenuation coefficient and buildup factors for engineering materials *American Nuclear Society,* La Grange Park, Illinois.

[22] Harima, Y. 1983 An approximation of gamma ray buildup factors by modified geometrical progression *Nucl. Sci. Eng*. 83, 299-309.

[23] Harima, Y. A historical review and current status of build-up factor calculations and applications. *Radiat. Phys. Chem.* 41, pp. 631-672, 1993.

[24] Manohara, S. R.; Hanagodimath, S. M.; Thind, K. S.; Gerward, L. On the effective atomic number and electron density: A comprehensive set of formulas for all types of materials and energies above 1 keV. *Nucl. Instr. And Meth. B* 2008, 266, 3906-3912.

[25] ICRU. *Radiation Quantities and Units Report 33 of the International Commission on Radiation Units and Measurements* (Bethesda, MD: ICRU) 1980.

[26] Gerward, L.; Guilbert, N.; Jensen, K. B.; Levring, H. X-ray absorption in matter. Reengineering XCOM. *Rad. Phys. and Chem.* 2001, 60, 23-24.

[27] Gerward, L.; Guilbert, N.; Jensen, K. B.; Levring, H. WinXCom- a program for calculating X-ray attenuation coefficients *Rad. Phys. and Chem.* 2004, 71, 653-654.

[28] Berger, M. J.; Hubbell, J. H. 1999 XCOM: Photon Cross Sections Database. Web Version 1.2, available at http:// physics.nist.gov/xcom, National Institute of Standards and Technology, Gaithersburg, MD 20899, USA, August 1999. Originally published as NBSIR 87-3597, XCOM: *Photon Cross Sections on a Personal Computer* (July 1987) 1987-1999.

[29] Chantler, C.T. Detailed Tabulation of Atomic Form Factors, Photoelectric Absorption and Scattering Cross Section, and Mass Attenuation Coefficients in the Vicinity of Absorption Edges in the Soft X-Ray (Z=30–36, Z=60–89, E=0.1 keV–10 keV), Addressing Convergence Issues of Earlier Work Detailed Tabulation of Atomic Form Factors, Photoelectric Absorption and Scattering Cross Section, and Mass Attenuation Coefficients in the Vicinity of Absorption Edges in the Soft X-Ray (Z=30–36, Z=60–89, E=0.1 keV–10 keV), Addressing Convergence Issues of Earlier Work. *J. Phys. Chem. Ref.* Data 2000, 29, 597.

[30] Asano, Y., Sakamoto, Y. 2007 Gamma Ray Buildup Factors for Heavy Concretes JAEData/Code 2007-006.

[31] Eisenhauer, C. M., Simmons, G. L. 1975 Point Isotropic Gamma Ray Buildup Factors in Concrete *Nucl. Sci. Eng.* 56.

In: Advances in Eye Research. Volume 1 ISBN 978-1-61324-169-1
Editor: W. L. Thomsen, pp. 93-111

Chapter IV

Uveitis in Juvenile Idiopathic Arthritis: Diagnosis and Treatment

Simone Appenzeller[1,*], Jozelio de Carvalho[2], Joyce Hisae Yamamoto[3] and Alexandre Wagner Silva de Souza[4]

[1]Rheumatology Division-Faculty Medical Science, State University of Campinas, Brazil

[2]Rheumatology Division University of São Paulo, School of Medicine, Brazil

[3]Department of Ophthalmology, University of São Paulo School of Medicine, Brazil

[4]Assistant physician at Universidade Federal de São Paulo, Brazil

---

* Correspondence: Dra. Simone Appenzeller, Disciplina de Reumatologia, Departamento de Clínica Médica Faculdade de Ciências Médicas, CP 6111 Universidade Estadual de Campinas – UNICAMP CEP 13083-970, Campinas, SP, Brasil. E-mail: appenzel@unicamp.br;

Grants:Dr Appenzeller: Fundação Apoio À Pesquisa Estado São Paulo-Brasil (FAPESP 2008/02917-0 and 2009/06049-6), Conselho Nacional Pesquisa Desenvolvimento-Brasil CNPq (300447/2009-4)

Abstract

Uveitis, an important manifestation of various autoimmune diseases and of some infectious disease, is a multifactorial disease. Children constitute 5-10% of the patients with uveitis seen at tertiary referral centers. The most common cause of anterior uveitis is idiopathic juvenile arthritis (JIA). The diagnosis and management of chronic pediatric uveitis can be particularly challenging, with an estimated 25-33% of childhood uveitis cases resulting in severe, life-long visual disability due to ocular complications such as cataract, band keratopathy, glaucoma and cystoid macular edema. Although infectious uveitis, once properly identified, may be successfully treated by addressing the inciting organism with specific therapy, the immune-mediated chronic forms of uveitis often provide more complex challenges in management. In addition uveitis associated with autoimmune diseases may be refractory unless the underlying systemic disease is adequately treated.

The aim of this chapter is to review uveitis in JIA and discuss possible treatment strategies.

Introduction

Intraocular inflammation affecting the uvea (uveitis) has varied infectious and non-infectious causes. In children, juvenile idiopathic arthritis (JIA) has been reported as the accompanying systemic manifestation in 41.5% to 81% of children with uveitis and in 75% to 95% of children with anterior uveitis [1, 2].

The special challenges in diagnosis and treatment of uveitis in children are well known to ophthalmologists: relatively few symptoms often lead to late presentation to eye specialists and, frequently, with already established pathology and significant decrease in visual acuity; difficulties in eliciting history, performing a review of systems, and examining children also pose special challenges. Visual losses in children due to uveitis remain a great concern. Despite aggressive treatment, some eyes may continue to lose vision.

In this chapter we will review clinical presentation, classification and treatment strategies of uveitis in juvenile idiopathic arthritis (JIA).

Terminology

Uveitis is a general term used to describe intraocular inflammation affecting the uvea. Uveal tract is the middle layer of the eye beneath the sclera [3, 4]. It consists of the iris, ciliary body and choroid. In clinical practice, the term uveitis, as used currently, is synonym of intraocular inflammation involving not only the uvea but extending to other ocular structures such as retina, vitreous, optic nerve and sclera [5-7].

Classification

When evaluating a patient with uveitis several clinical characteristics may help to identify the etiology, including: [1] anatomic location of the inflammation; [2] disease course; [3] presence of a causative infection (e.g., syphilis or Lyme disease); [4] presence of an associated systemic disorder (e.g., sarcoidosis or a spondyloarthropathy); and [5] presence of a morphologic syndrome (e.g., birdshot chorioretinitis [BSCR]) [7, 8].

Classification is based on Standardization of Uveitis Nomenclature Working Group [8] (Table 1). The combination of these clinical characteristics is essential to establish a correct diagnosis [5].

Epidemiology

Children constitute 3-10% of patients with uveitis seen at tertiary referral centers [9, 10]. Annual incidence rates of pediatric uveitis in North America and Europe is estimated to be 4.3 to 6.9/100,000; lower than estimates for adults [9, 11]. The same population-based studies estimated the prevalence of uveitis in children to be approximately 30 cases in 100,000 [12, 13]. In recent series, proportion of children with anterior uveitis varies from 9.4% to 47% [14]. Juvenile idiopathic arthritis-associated uveitis accounts for approximately 75% of all pediatric anterior uveitis cases and is the most common systemic cause of uveitis of childhood [15]. Infectious causes of uveitis are observed among 5-33% of children in recent publications [14]. Although frequently associated with an underlying systemic disease, e.g. juvenile idiopathic arthritis (JIA) [16], a significant proportion of uveitis are labeled idiopathic.

Table 1. Classification of uveitis

Classification	Characteristics
Anatomic	
Anterior	iritis, iridocyclitis
Intermediate	cyclitis, vitritis, pars planitis
Posterior	focal, multifocal choroiditis, retinitis
Diffuse	panuveitis
Age (yr)	
0-16	
16-40	
>40	
Course	
Acute	sudden onset and limited duration
Recurrent	repeated episodes separated by periods of inactivity
Chronic	without treatment $\geq$ 3 months of duration persisten uveitis with relapse in < 3 months after discontinuing treatment
Onset	
Sudden	
Insidious	
Duration	
Limited	$\leq$ 3 months duration
Persistent	>3 months duration
Laterality	
Unilateral	
Bilateral	
Etiology	
Infeccious	
Non infectious	
Or	
Isolated ocular disease	
Associated with systemic disease	

Adapted from The Standardization of Uveitis Nomenclature (SUN) Working Group. [8].

Physiopathology

The eye is an immune privileged organ and enjoys a special relationship with the immune system. Immune privilege comprises a set of mechanisms observed in certain organs such as the brain, the eye, and the liver, that control inflammation and prevent wide spread destruction of tissue even during the event of an immune response [6]. An efficient blood–retina barrier, active local inhibition by soluble and surface-bound molecules that inhibit activation and function of adaptive and innate immune cells are involved in the protection from local inflammatory responses [6,7, 17].

Both Th1 and Th17 are involved in the pathogenesis of uveitis [17]. Once T cells that recognize uveitogenic epitopes are activated they migrate to the eye and initiate a cascade of events leading to the destruction of the photoreceptor layer and loss of vision [6]. Any activated T cell can penetrate the retina, however, only cells recognizing uveitogenic epitopes will remain in the retina after 12 h [18]. Through the secretion of various cytokines that induce expression of adhesion molecules and MHC class II these cells contribute to the blood–retinal barrier breakdown, allowing the recruitment of other T cells as well as monocytes and polymorphonuclear cells from the blood [6, 7].

Cytokines have also an important role in the development of uveitis. Interleukin (IL)-1 has been shown important in the breakdown of the retinal-blood barrier and as an enhancer of inflammation to the same extent as IL-7 [19]. IL-2 has been shown to be important both in the activation and proliferation of uveitogenic T cells [6, 20]. IL-12 family of cytokines (IL-12, IL-23 and IL-27) plays a central role in the development of inflammatory diseases that require IFN-γ synthesis [6]. The production of IFN-γ and TNF has been often associated with autoimmune uveitis and used as a marker of disease development and severity [6, 21-23].

Juvenile Idiopathic Arthritis (JIA) Uveitis

JIA is defined as arthritis of unknown etiology that begins before the age of 16 years and persists for at least 6 weeks. Several subgroups of JIA are well recognized and they differ in clinical manifestations, prognosis, specific autoimmune features, and genetic determinants [24]. The International League of Associations for Rheumatology devised a new classification system, revised in 2001 [25], and divided JIA into 7 subtypes, which are mutually exclusive: systemic arthritis, oligoarthritis (persistent and extended subtypes), polyarthritis (both rheumatoid factor positive and negative), psoriatic arthritis, enthesitis-related arthritis, and undifferentiated arthritis [11, 26] (Table 2). In populations of European ancestry, oligoarthritis is the most common subtype, comprising 50-70% of cases; polyarthritis occurs in about 30% and systemic onset disease and enthesitis-related arthritis in about 5% each of children with JIA [27]. Uveitis is associated with anti-nuclear antibody (ANA) positivity, young age at onset of arthritis (< 6 years) and female sex [27].

The most frequent extra-articular manifestation of JIA is an insidious asymptomatic anterior uveitis with a chronic disease course, which has no comparable counterpart in adults [24]. This chronic uveitis occurs in about 20% of JIA patients with oligoarthritis, particularly in ANA-positive girls with early onset oligoarthritis [28]. It occurs less frequently (in 5–10%) in patients with RF-negative polyarthritis and virtually never in patients with RF-positive polyarthritis and in systemic onset disease [28, 29]. In most cases both eyes are affected, either simultaneously or within a few months of each other [28]. It is uncommon in initially unilateral uveitis for the inflammation to develop in the other eye more than a year from the onset of the process [28]. In a majority of cases uveitis is non granulomatous with a flare and cells in the anterior chamber [28]. Sometimes an exacerbation of uveitis causes redness and discomfort in a patient with formerly symptomless uveitis [28].

Another form of uveitis observed is the more acute and clearly symptomatic anterior uveitis, which has its counterpart in HLA B27-associated acute anterior uveitis in adults. Such patients are typically negative for antinuclear antibodies (ANA) and RF [28]. Acute anterior uveitis is often found in connection with enthesitis-related arthritis in children positive for HLA B27, most of whom are boys at the age of 10 or more, who may later develop spondyloarthropathy [28]. Patients with psoriatic arthritis not infrequently have chronic uveitis, although no precise figures are available due to the rarity of this condition [28].

Uveitis is rarely (< than 10% of cases) diagnosed prior to the onset of arthritis [28, 29]. However, it is quite often detected at the first ophthalmologic consultation in the early phases of arthritis [28]. Most frequently, uveitis is diagnosed during the first 7 years of arthritis, but it has been described to occur 20 years after the onset of disease [28].

Table 2. The Subtypes of JIA and prevalence of uveitis. Adapted from Zierhut et al [67]

Subtypes of JIA	Prevalence of uveitis	Marker
Systemic arthritis	Rare	
Oligoarthritis a) persistent b) extended	15-40%, asymptomatic	ANA 70-90%
Polyarthritis, rheumatoid factor-negative	5-10%, asymptomatic	ANA 30%
Polyarthritis, rheumatoid factor-positive	Rare	RF
Psoriatic arthritis	<20%, asymptomatic and symptomatic	
Enthesitis-related arthritis	~10%, symptomatic	HLA B27
Other forms of arthritis	Rare	None

ANA: Antinuclear antibodies; RF: Rheumatoid factor.

Although the activities of joint and eye inflammation may parallel each other, they are in fact more commonly independent [28, 30]. In addition the presence of uveitis does not foretell the long-term articular prognosis of oligoarthritis [31]. On the other hand, in a series of 372 children with recently diagnosed JIA, clinical and laboratory parameters showed more active arthritis in patients with uveitis than in those without it. Clinical remission of arthritis was also significantly less frequent in patients with uveitis than in those without [32].

Follow-up studies of JIA-associated uveitis are difficult to be performed, because the children change to adult clinic during the disease course. There is anecdotal evidence indicating that uveitis in adult age can be quiescent while arthritis continues active [28]. However, there are no studies dealing with the relationship between arthritis and uveitis in adult age [28].

Visual impairment has been shown to be as high as 40% of which 10% being blind.

Uveitis Screening

The American Academy of Pediatrics published formal guidelines for the frequency of ophthalmologic screening for patients with JIA in 1993 and 2006 [33]. Age of onset, a positive ANA titer, and subtype of JIA, and disease duration were important parameters for screening [11]. Patients less than age 6 years in the ANA positive pauciarticular and polyarticular groups were designated high risk to be screened every 3 to 4 months, whereas patients with systemic JIA were designated low risk regardless of age of onset and were to be screened annually [11, 33]. All others were designated moderate risk to be screened every 6 months [11, 33]. It may also be important to continue uveitis screening yearly late into adulthood since rare cases of uveitis can develop decades after the arthritis [35].

Uveitis Differential Diagnosis

The JIA associated uveitis should be differentiate from uveitis of other etiologies such as trauma, infection or another non-infectious disease [11]. Blunt trauma to the eye may produce pain, redness, and photophobia several days later [10, 36].

For anterior infectious uveitis, herpes virus family, syphilis, tuberculosis, and, less frequently, Lyme disease and cat-scratch disease, should be discarded [36]. In addition to JIA, anterior uveitis also occurs in 60% of patients with sarcoidosis, and is usually chronic with minimal symptoms though acute symptoms may develop [11]. Although uncommon, intermediate, posterior and panuveitis have been described in sarcoidosis.

Other conditions to consider in the differential diagnosis of uveitis in children include tubulointerstitial nephritis and uveitis syndrome, Kawasaki arteritis, Behçet´s disease, and Vogt-Koyanagi-Harada disease [11].

Treatment

The goal of treatment is to control ocular inflammation, prevent or minimize the sight-threatening complications, and to avoid recurrence [27]. JIA patients with uveitis should be referred to an experienced ophthalmologist for treatment and follow-up. For severe uveitis, treatment should be multiprofessional, with close cooperation between ophthalmologists and pediatric rheumatologists [27]. The most important steps are awareness of the occurrence of asymptomatic uveitis in JIA, close follow-up to allow an early diagnosis and prompt treatment [27, 37-39].

The management of patients with JIA-associated uveitis should be approached in a step-wise progression beginning with topical steroids and mydriatics, progressing to regional steroids, systemic NSAIDs, systemic steroids, immunosuppressive agents, and biologics.

Topical and Regional (Peri or Intraocular) Corticosteroids

Topical corticosteroid, such as prednisolone acetate 1% or dexamethasone 0.1%, is the mainstay of therapy for anterior uveitis [11]. Drops may be administered hourly for severe inflammation [11, 40]. Glaucoma and cataract are frequent side effects of topical steroid therapy in children with JIA [11, 41,42]. Cataract in children may lead to the development of amblyopia and require prompt surgical removal.

Most patients would respond to this initial treatment. The presence of vitreous cells, severe disease, or chronic inflammation increases the risk for cystoid macular edema. The decision to use regional corticosteroids depends on the patient´s response to topical therapy and/or the presence of posterior segment involvement. Monocular involvement also weighs in more toward regional corticosteroid use whereas bilaterality may favor the use of systemic corticosteroid.

Mydriatic and Cycloplegic Agents

Mydriasis and cycloplegia are important therapeutic adjuncts for uveitis. Topical agents relieve ciliary spasm and pain that often accompany iridocyclitis, and prevent the development of posterior synechiae [11, 40].

Systemic Corticosteroids

Systemic corticosteroids are recommended for severe, usually bilateral, disease, or for patients who develop significant side effects of topical agents [11, 40, 41]. Oral prednisone (1mg/kg/day for 2-4 weeks) may be given to rapidly control inflammation [11, 42]. Side-effects include e.g. weight gain, mood changes, growth restriction, hypertension, avascular necrosis [11, 40].

Immunosuppressants

Immunosuppressive treatment should be considered for children with JIA-related uveitis who have uncontrolled uveitis despite prolonged high-dose topical treatment, especially if they already have synechiae [43].

Methotrexate

Methotrexate is the most common disease-modifying agent used to treat active arthritis in JIA [11]. It may also control uveitis. Administration varies according to body surface, but ranges between 7.5 to 30 mg weekly. It may be given orally or subcutaneous, the latter presenting enhanced efficacy with doses above 20mg/week [11].

Cyclosporine

Several studies have shown that cyclosporine effectively controls uveitis and reduces steroid dosing [44, 45]. Side effects include arterial hypertension and renal toxicity. These studies indicated a good tolerability and efficacy; cyclosporine should be considered as a second line therapy, especially in patients intolerant to methotrexate [11].

Azathioprine

In a retrospective study of 41 JIA patients with uveitis, azathioprine was used alone or in combination with other immunosuppressant drugs [46]. At 1 year, uveitis inactivity was achieved in 13/17 (76.5%) patients by using azathioprine as systemic monotherapy and in 5/9 (56.6%) as combination therapy. The authors concluded that azathioprine may be reconsidered in the stepladder approach for the treatment of JIA-associated uveitis. The addition of azathioprine may also be beneficial for patients not responding properly to methotrexate [46].

Mycophenolate Mofetil

Small case series studies have demonstrated the efficacy of mycophenolate mofetil in JIA-associated uveitis with little or no side effects [4, 47, 48]. However, further studies of larger cohorts are indicated to assess the use of mycophenolate mofetil in JIA-associated uveitis.

Chlorambucil

Although a few studies [49, 50] have used chlorambucil in refractory uveitis associated with JIA, the toxicity profile of chlorambucil suggests it should be used very cautiously. The primary side effects include bone marrow suppression, gonadal toxicity and malignancy [11].

Tumor Necrosis Factor-α Inhibitors

Etanercept

Several studies, including prospective trials have analyzed the effect of etanercept on uveitis in JIA patients. Etanercept may be useful for methotrexate refractory JIA-associated uveitis, in doses 0.8mg/kg/week. However, the high rates of recurrence and development of uveitis while on etanercept therapy suggest that it may not be the most effective therapy for JIA-associated uveitis [11, 51-53].

Infliximab

In small studies infliximab has been shown to be effective for refractory uveitis in JIA. Recommended doses are 5 to 10 mg/kg every 2 to 4 weeks and then every 4 to 8 weeks for maintenance. Studies have suggested that infliximab is effective in treating JIA-associated uveitis, especially in severe and refractory cases [11, 54-57].

Adalimumab

Several studies, including prospective trials have analyzed the effect of adalimumab on uveitis in JIA patients [58-60]. Adalimumab is a potential treatment option in JIA-associated uveitis, even in patients non-responsive to previous other anti-TNF therapy [58-60].

Other Biologic Options

Abatacept

A selective co-stimulation modulator that inhibits T-cell activation by binding to CD80 and CED86, thereby blocking CD28 interaction. CD28 interaction provides a signal needed for full T-cell activation. Recently, small case series report the use of abatacept (10 mg/kg monthly) in refractory JIA uveitis with sustained improvement [61, 62]. These results provide new insights into a possible indication of abatacept for the treatment of JIA uveitis [62].

JIA-associated Uveitis Complications

JIA-associated uveitis result in significant impairment of visual acuity as a consequence of structural ocular complications such as cataract (10-84%), band keratopathy (0-70%), glaucoma (11-30%), hypotony (0-17%) and macular pathology [27, 39]. The cumulative incidence of vision loss in these patients points to a frequency of blindness of 24% at three years [63].

Complicated cataract develops secondary to severe inflammation in the anterior chamber [26]. In addition prolonged systemic use of corticosteroids even in the absence of uveitis is a risk factor for the formation of posterior subcapsular cataract [27, 64]. Modern ophthalmic surgery with microsurgical progress in cataract extraction has improved the prognosis of JIA-associated uveitis patients with complicated cataract, but intraocular lens implantation remains controversial [27]. Complete control of inflammation 3 months prior to surgery is related to better post-operative prognosis.

Longstanding intraocular inflammation may cause band keratopathy, where an accumulation of calcium is seen at the level of Bowman's membrane in the cornea [27]. This clouded cornea can be cleared by chelating agents or excimer laser.

Secondary glaucoma is another sight-threatening complication of JIA-associated uveitis. Blockage of the aqueous outflow due to inflammation, peripheral anterior synechiae, pupillary block due to posterior synechiae and secondary angle closure, in addition to topical corticosteroid treatment are common causes of secondary glaucoma in JIA [27]. Secondary glaucoma is often refractory to medial treatment and glaucoma implant devices is a therapeutic option.

Chronic anterior uveitis in JIA may spread to the posterior segment of the eye, causing accumulation of cells and protein in the vitreous (vitritis), multicystic collection of fluid within macula (cystoid macular edema) or disc edema. Cystoid macular edema is an important cause of visual impairment in such cases. Because it can only rarely be confirmed by fluorescein angiography, the evaluation is based on funduscopy. Loss of foveal reflex and a wet, glistening reflex in the foveal area are the first signs, and this may progress to the cystoid pattern in a few weeks or months [27, 65].

Severe uveitis can rarely result in epiretinal membranes, retinal detachment, and finally in hypotony and phthisis bulbi. In these cases the prognosis is frequently poor [27].

Complications from JIA-associated uveitis are significantly more likely in patients with uveitis at initial presentation and in those with more severe ocular disease at onset [27]. Risk factors include male sex, and decreased time between development of arthritis [27, 66]. Despite aggressive treatment with a variety of agents 96.6% still developed at least 1 complication [27].

Thus, it is important to monitor patients with JIA according to the guidelines to screen especially for asymptomatic uveitis. This screening should be perfomed also in adult patients with JIA.

References

[1] Kanski JJ. Shu-Shin GA. Systemc uveitis syndromes in childhood: an analysis of 340 cases. *Ophthalmology* 1984;91:1247-52.

[2] Tugal-Tutkun I, Havrlikova K, Power WJ et al. Changing patterns in uveitis of childhood. *Ophthalmology* 1996; 103:375-83.

[3] Pato E, Muñoz-Fernández S, Francisco F, Abad MA, Maese J, Ortiz A, Carmona L; Uveitis Working Group from Spanish Society of Rheumatology. Systematic Review on the Effectiveness of Immunosuppressants and Biological Therapies in the Treatment of Autoimmune Posterior Uveitis. *Semin Arthritis Rheum.* 2010 Jul 23. [Epub ahead of print]

[4] Muñoz-Fernández S, Martín-Mola E. Uveitis. *Best Pract Res Clin Rheumatol.* 2006;20:487-505.

[5] Bloch-Michel E & Nussenblatt RB. International uveitis study group recommendations for the evaluation of intraocular inflammatory disease. *American Journal of Ophthalmology* 1987; 103: 234–235.

[6] Vallochi AL, Commodaro AG, Schwartzman JP, Belfort R Jr, Rizzo LV. The role of cytokines in the regulation of ocular autoimmune inflammation. *Cytokine Growth Factor Rev.* 2007;18:135-41.

[7] Zamecki KJ, Jabs DA. HLA typing in uveitis: use and misuse. *Am J Ophthalmol.* 2010;149:189-193.

[8] The Standardization of Uveitis Nomenclature (SUN) Working Group. Standardization of uveitis nomenclature for reporting clinical data. Results of the First International Workshop. *Am J Ophthalmol* 2005;140:509 –516.

[9] Holland GN, Stiehm ER. Special considerations in the evaluation and management of uveitis in children. *Am J Ophthalmol.* 2003;135:867–878.

[10] Kimura SJ, Hogan MJ. Uveitis in children: analysis of 274 cases. *Trans Am Ophthalmol Soc* 1964; 62: 173–192.

[11] Wright T, Cron RQ. Pediatric rheumatology for the adult rheumatologist II: uveitis in juvenile idiopathic arthritis. *J Clin Rheumatol.* 2007;13:205-10.

[12] Paivonsalo-Hietanen T, J. Tuominen and K.M. Saari, Uveitis in children: population-based study in Finland. *Acta Ophthalmol Scand* 2000; 78 : 84–88.

[13] Darrell RW, Wagener HP and Kurland LT. Epidemiology of uveitis. *Arch Ophthalmol* 1962; 68: 100–112.

[14] Kump LI, Cervantes-Castañeda RA, Androudi SN, Foster CS. Analysis of Pediatric Uveitis Cases at a Tertiary Referral Center. *OPhthalmology* 2005; 112:1287-1292.

[15] Simonini G, Cantarini L, Bresci C, Lorusso M, Galeazzi M, Cimaz R. Current therapeutic approaches to autoimmune chronic uveitis in children. *Autoimmun Rev.* 2010;9:674-83

[16] Punzi L, Furlan A, Podswiadek M, Gava A, Valente M, De Marchi M, et al. Clinical and genetic aspects of Blau syndrome: a 25-year follow-up of one family and a literature review. *Autoimmun Rev* 2009;8:228–32.

[17] Caspi R. Autoimmunity in the immune privileged eye: pathogenic and regulatory T cells. *Immunol Res.* 2008;42: 41-50.

[18] Prendergast RA, Iliff CE, Coskuncan NM, Caspi RR, Sartani G, Tarrant TK, et al. T cell traffic and the inflammatory response in experimental autoimmune uveoretinitis. *Invest Ophthalmol Vis Sci* 1998;39:754.

[19] Luna JD, Chan CC, Derevjanik NL, Mahlow J, Chiu C, Peng B, et al. Blood–retinal barrier (BRB) breakdown in experimental autoimmune uveoretinitis: comparison with vascular endothelial growth factor, tumor necrosis factor alpha, and interleukin-1beta-mediated breakdown. *J Neurosci Res* 1997;49:268.

[20] Su SB, Silver PB, Grajewski RS, Agarwal RK, Tang J, Chan CC, et al. Essential role of the MyD88 pathway, but nonessential roles of TLRs 2,4 and 9, in the adjuvant effect promoting Th1-mediated autoimmunity. *J Immunol* 2005;175:6303.

[21] Jones LS, Rizzo LV, Agarwal RK, Tarrant TK, Chan CC, Wiggert B, et al. IFN-gamma-deficient mice develop experimental autoimmune uveitis in the context of a deviant effector response. *J Immunol* 1997;158:5997.

[22] Sun B, Rizzo LV, Sun SH, Chan CC, Wiggert B, Wilder RL, et al. Genetic susceptibility to experimental autoimmune uveitis involves more than a predisposition to generate a T helper-1-like or a T helper-2-like response. *J Immunol* 1997;159:1004.

[23] Rizzo LV. The subsets of T helper cells involved in the development of experimental autoimmune uveoretinitis. *Ophthalmol McGill* 1994;6:5.

[24] Sabri K, Saurenmann RK, Silverman ED, Levin AV. Course, complications, and outcome of juvenile arthritis-related uveitis. *J AAPOS.* 2008;12:539-45.

[25] Petty RE, Southwood TR, Manners P, et al. International League of Associations for Rheumatology classification of juvenile idiopathic arthritis: second revision, Edmonton, 2001. *J Rheumatol.* 2004;31:390–392.

[26] Jabs DA, Nussenblatt RB, Rosenbaum JT. Standardization of uveitis nomenclature for reporting clinical data: Results of the First International Workshop. *Am J Ophthalmol* 2005;140:509-16.

[27] Kotaniemi K, Savolainen A, Karma A, Aho K. Recent Advances in uveitis of juvenile idiopathic arthritis. *Surv Ophthalmol* 2003; 48:489-502

[28] Kotaniemi K, Savolainen A, Karma A, Aho K. Recent advances in uveitis of juvenile idiopathic arthritis. *Surv Ophthalmol.* 2003;48:489-502.

[29] Edelsten C, Lee V, Bentley CR, et al: An evaluation of baseline risk factors predicting severity in juvenile idiopathic arthritis associated uveitis and other chronic anterior uveitis in early childhood. *Br J Ophthalmol* 2002; 86:51–6.

[30] Rosenberg AM, Oen KG: The relationship between ocular and articular disease activity in children with juvenile rheumatoid arthritis and associated uveitis. *Arthritis Rheum* 1986; 29:797–800.

[31] Cimaz RG, Fink CW: The articular prognosis of pauciarticular onset juvenile arthritis is not influenced by the presence of uveitis. *J Rheumatol* 1996; 23:357–9.

[32] Kotaniemi K, Kotaniemi A, Savolainen A: Uveitis as amarker of active arthritis in 372 patients with juvenile idiopathic seronegative oligoarthritis or polyarthritis. *Clin Exp Rheumatol* 2002; 20:109–12.

[33] American academy of pediatrics section on rheumatology and section on ophthalmology: guidelines for ophthalmologic examinations in children with juvenile rheumatoid arthritis. *Pediatrics* 1993;92:295–296.

[34] Cassidy J, Kivlin J, Lindsley C, et al. Ophthalmologic examinations in children with juvenile rheumatoid arthritis. *Pediatrics* 2006;117:1843–1845.

[35] Kotaniemi K. Late onset uveitis in juvenile-type chronic polyarthritis controlled with prednisolone, cyclosporin A and methotrexate. *Clin ExpRheumatol. 1998*;16:469–471.

[36] Patel H, Goldstein D. Pediatric uveitis. *Pediatr Clin North Am.* 2003; 50:125–136.

[37] Dollfus H: Eye involvement in childrens rheumatic diseases. *Baillieres Clin Rheumatol* 1998; 12:309–28.

[38] Nguyen QD, Foster CS: Saving the vision of children with juvenile rheumatoid arthritis-associated uveitis. *JAMA* 1998; 280:1133–4.

[39] Waheed NK, Miserocchi E, Foster CS: Ocular concerns in juvenile rheumatoid arthritis. *Int Ophthalmol Clin* 2001; 41:223–34.

[40] Smith JR. Management of uveitis in pediatric patients: special considerations. *Paediatr Drugs*. 2002;4:183–189.

[41] Kwok AK, Lam DS, Ng JS, et al. Ocular-hypertensive response to topical steroids in children. *Ophthalmology*. 1997;104:2112–2116.

[42] *Saurenmann RK Arthritis & Rhuematism 2007*;56:647-57.

[43] Gerloni V, Cimaz R, Gattinara M, et al. Efficacy and safety profile of cyclosporin A in the treatment of juvenile chronic (idiopathic) arthritis. Results of a 10-year prospective study. *Rheumatology (Oxford*). 2001; 40:907–913.

[44] Kilmartin DJ, Forrester JV, Dick AD. Cyclosporin A therapy in refractory non-infectious childhood uveitis. *Br J Ophthalmol.* 1998;82:737–742.

[45] Goebel JC, Roesel M, Heinz C, Michels H, Ganser G, Heiligenhaus A. Azathioprine as a treatment option for uveitis in patients with juvenile idiopathic arthritis. Br J Ophthalmol. 2010 Jun 28. [Epub ahead of print]

[46] Thorne JE, Jabs DA, Qazi FA, et al. Mycophenolate mofetil therapy for inflammatory eye disease. *Ophthalmology*. 2005;112:1472–1477.

[47] Baltatzis S, Tufail F, Yu EN, et al. Mycophenolate mofetil as an immunomodulatory agent in the treatment of chronic ocular inflammatory disorders. *Ophthalmology*. 2003;110:1061–1065.

[48] Palmer RG, Kanski JJ, Ansell BM. Chlorambucil in the treatment of intractable uveitis associated with juvenile chronic arthritis. *J Rheumatol.* 1985;12:967–970.

[49] Miserocchi E, Baltatzis S, Ekong A, et al. Efficacy and safety of chlorambucil in intractable noninfectious uveitis: the Massachusetts eye and ear infirmary experience. *Ophthalmology*. 2002;109:137–142.

[50] Reiff A, Takei S, Sadeghi S, et al. Etanercept therapy in children with treatment-resistant uveitis. *Arthritis Rheum.* 2001;44:1411–1415.

[51] Reiff A. Long-term outcome of etanercept therapy in children with treatment-refractory uveitis. *Arthritis Rheum.* 2003; 48:2079 –2080.

[52] Smith JA, Thompson DJ, Whitcup SM, et al. A randomized, placebo controlled, double-masked clinical trial of etanercept for the treatment

of uveitis associated with juvenile idiopathic arthritis. *Arthritis Rheum.* 2005;53:18 –23.

[53] Richards JC, Tay-Kearney ML, Murray K, et al. Infliximab for juvenile idiopathic arthritis-associated uveitis. *Clin Experiment Ophthalmol.* 2005;33:461– 468.

[54] Saurenmann RK, Levin AV, Rose JB, et al. Tumour necrosis factor alpha inhibitors in the treatment of childhood uveitis. *Rheumatology* (Oxford). 2006;45:982–989.

[55] Rajaraman RT, Kimura Y, Li S, et al. Retrospective case review of pediatric patients with uveitis treated with infliximab. *Ophthalmology.* 2006;113:308 –314.

[56] Kahn P, Weiss M, Imundo LF, et al. Favorable response to high-dose infliximab for refractory childhood uveitis. *Ophthalmology.* 2006;113: 860–864.

[57] Biester S, Deuter C, Michels H, Haefner R, Kuemmerle-Deschner J, Doycheva D, Zierhut M. Adalimumab in the therapy of uveitis in childhood. *Br J Ophthalmol.* 2007;91:319-24.

[58] Chen YF, Jobanputra P, Barton P, Jowett S, Bryan S, Clark W, Fry-Smith A, Burls A. A systematic review of the effectiveness of adalimumab, etanercept and infliximab for the treatment of rheumatoid arthritis in adults and an economic evaluation of their cost-effectiveness. *Health Technol Assess.* 2006;10, 1-229.

[59] Tynjälä P, Kotaniemi K, Lindahl P, Latva K, Aalto K, Honkanen V, Lahdenne P. Adalimumab in juvenile idiopathic arthritis-associated chronic anterior uveitis. *Rheumatology (Oxford).* 2008;47:339-44.

[60] Kenawy N, Cleary G, Mewar D, Beare N, Chandna A, Pearce I. Abatacept: a potential therapy in refractory cases of juvenile idiopathic arthritis-associated uveitis. *Graefes Arch Clin Exp Ophthalmol.* 2010 Oct 5. [Epub ahead of print]

[61] Zulian F, Balzarin M, Falcini F, Martini G, Alessio M, Cimaz R, Cimino L, Zannin ME. Abatacept for severe anti-tumor necrosis factor alpha refractory juvenile idiopathic arthritis-related uveitis. *Arthritis Care Res (Hoboken).* 2010 ;62:821-5.

[62] Thorne JE, Woreta F, Kedhar SR, Dunn JP, Jabs DA. Juvenile idiopathic arthritis-associated uveitis: incidence of ocular complications and visual acuity loss. *Am J Ophthalmol.* 2007 May;143(5):840-846.

[63] Urban RC Jr, Cotlier E: Corticosteroid-induced cataracts. *Surv Ophthalmol* 1986; 31:102–10.

[64] Vesterdal E, Sury B: Iridocyclitis and bandshaped corneal opacity in juvenile rheumatoid arthritis. *Acta Ophthalmol* 1950; 28:321–37.

[65] Kalinina Ayuso V, Ten Cate HA, van der Does P, Rothova A, de Boer JH. Male gender as a risk factor for complications in uveitis associated with juvenile idiopathic arthritis. *Am J Ophthalmol* 2010;149:994–999.

[66] Zierhut M, MIchels H, Stübiger N, Besch D, Deuter C, Hellgenhaus A. *Uveitis in Children Int Ophthalmol Clin* 2005; 45:135-156.

In: Advances in Eye Research. Volume 1 ISBN 978-1-61324-169-1
Editor: W. L. Thomsen, pp. 113-129

Chapter V

Retinal Vasculitis in Rheumatic Diseases: Unseen Burden

***Sofia Androudi*[1], *Evangelia Tsironi*[1], *Leila Kump*[2] *and Shree K. Kurup*[3]**

[1]Department of Ophthalmology, University of Thessalia, Larissa, Greece
[2]Department of Ophthalmology, University of Kansas School of Medicine, Prairie Village, Kansas, USA
[3]Department of Ophthalmology and Internal Medicine, Wake Forest University, Winston-Salem, NC. 27157, USA

Abstract

Retinal vascular inflammation, a potentially blinding condition (herein: retinal vasculitis - RV) is commonly associated with a heterogeneous group of diseases characterized by systemic inflammatory cell infiltration and/or necrosis of blood vessel walls. RV may arise as a primary or secondary disorder (rheumatoid arthritis, Wegener's granulomatosis, polyarteritis nodosa) or it can be secondary to an underlying collagen disease, systemic refection or malignancy. Depending on the type of RV, it can be potentially blinding; in the short or long term. Early diagnosis is the key to successful treatment and better prognosis.

However, early diagnosis can be difficult, because these conditions usually present with non-specific visual symptoms for a long period before diagnostic manifestations occur.

RV can be detected clinically (often accompanied by uveitis, scleritis, macular edema) or revealed on fluorescein fundus angiography, even if minimal clinical and ophthalmologic signs of retinal vessel inflammation are present. Therefore the retina should be examined in warranted patients with rheumatic disease, since retinal vasculitis may be asymptomatic at the beginning (peripheral retinal disease). RV can also represent one of the possible extra-articular manifestations of the rheumatic disease. Rheumatologists should be familiar with the ocular manifestations of these disorders, since they may not only be sight threatening, but more importantly, could be the presenting – or even the very first manifestations of active, potentially lethal systemic disease in a patient with non specific rheumatologic presentation.

I. Introduction

The burden of uveitis is significant enough to classify it as the most blinding entity after diabetes and glaucoma in the younger productive population [1]. The diagnosis of retinal vasculitis (RV), a subtype of uveitic disease often remains challenging because of the wide spectrum of its clinical and pathological manifestations, the lack of specific signs and symptoms, and the absence of reliable tests. Blood vessel inflammation and necrosis are the main pathological features associated with vasculitis. Necrosis of the endothelial layers leads to destruction and occlusion of vessels, with subsequent poor perfusion and ischemia of the end organ, in this case the eye. The clinical features of RV vary immensely and are dependent on the site, type, size and distribution of the vessels involved by the inflammatory response as well as the underlying systemic disease.

Vasculitis syndromes may be initial presentation of systemic immune mediated disorders. [2] It is important for the rheumatologist to remember that the vasculitic process is not limited (in the eye) to the retinal circulation. Ocular manifestations of systemic vasculitides can present in many forms, including conjunctivitis, episcleritis, scleritis, peripheral ulcerative keratitis (PUK) and uveitis. [2] Prompt recognition and association of ocular symptoms with a diagnosis of systemic vasculitis is critical to prevent permanent visual sequelae. The goal of this review is to present and discuss the clinical features of retinal vasculitis in the more common rheumatic diseases. Our goal is to provide interested clinicians with an aid in the prompt diagnosis of these conditions and provide a skeleton framework to further therapeutic approaches.

II. Retinal Vasculitis in Rheumatic Diseases

The ophthalmic examination can be vital in the diagnosis and treatment of rheumatic diseases with evidence of systemic vasculitis. The ophthalmologist will be involved in the evaluation of patients with vasculitis who present for the first time with ocular symptoms or who are referred with a known diagnosis of rheumatic disease for an ophthalmic examination and determination of disease activity and extension. In patients presenting for the first time with only ocular symptoms, the role of the ophthalmologist is crucial in making a diagnosis or providing the internist with the information necessary to create a focused differential diagnosis and treatment plan. Rheumatologists have attempted to include end-organ involvement information, in an effort to create a universal scoring system that could be used to diagnose and treat these conditions.

A complete ophthalmic examination should include a detailed medical history with history of the present illness, past medical history and a thorough review of systems, in addition to the ocular history. The patient's previous history of infections, neoplasms, drug-sensitivity and rheumatological diseases, must be especially carefully elicited, to distinguish between primary and secondary vasculitis. The ophthalmic examination must be complemented with the systemic examination and timed appropriately.

III. Manifestations of Retinal Vasculitis in Rheumatic Diseases

A. Symptoms of Retinal Vasculitis

1. Asymptomatic (common)
2. Blurred vision (due to macular edema or ischemia)
3. Decreased vision

4. Inability to read at near
5. Improved distance vision in nearsighted patients (due to macular edema causing hyperopia)
6. Visual Field deficits

B. Signs of Retinal Vasculitis

1. Cotton-wool spots
2. Retinal hemorrhage: dot, blot, flame-shaped
3. Preretinal hemorrhage
4. Microaneurysms
5. Macular Edema
6. Focal narrowing of retinal vasculature
7. Arterial occlusion with focal deposits
8. Central/ Branch retinal arterial occlusion with cherry red spot
9. Central/ Branch venous occlusion
10. Retinal neovascularization
11. Anterior segment ischemia
12. Vitreous hemorrhage
13. Neovascular or hemorrhagic glaucoma
14. Hypertensive changes (arteriolar narrowing, hard exudates, flame hemorrhages, optic disk edema)
15. Optic disk vasculitis and neuritis

IV. Diagnostic Ancillary Ophthalmic Investigations

A. Fluorescein Angiography (FFA)

Besides clinical examination patients with RV should preferably be evaluated; prior to institution of systemic therapy, at a uveitis center. Funduscopic signs of vasculitis include retinal arterial sheathing. A fundus angiogram using intravenous dye fluorescein (mw: 332) adds great value in understanding the extent of retinal involvement. This will help also resolve the confusion between vasculopathy (as in hypertensive or lupus vasculopathy: no inflammation, only endothelial dysfunction) and establish a baseline. The leakage of the dye leads to progressive retinal vessel wall hyperfluorecence detected by special filters in the camera in active retinal disease. Inflammation of the retinal vasculature may lead to focal leakage from the retinal capillaries and arterioles. Vasculitis of the optic nerve may lead to optic nerve head swelling and subsequent ischemic optic neuropathy.

B. Optical Coherence Tomography (OCT)

OCT utilizing non invasive near infra red photography was initially used in ophthalmology and its use has extended into medicine. This technique examines retina in a cross-section, simulating histopathology studies. This imaging modality can reveal macular edema (as thickened retina) or explain poor vision (atrophic retina) in retinal vasculitis patients. This investigative modality can also be easily incorporated into rheumatologic study protocols.

V. Typical Model of Retinal Vasculitis as Seen in SLE

The most recognized ocular manifestation of SLE is lupus retinopathy [3-4]. In this manuscript, SLE associated RV (SLE-RV) will serve as the prototypal model and other entities would be characterized by comparison to this model. SLE-RV, a potentially bilaterally blinding condition is considered an important marker of disease activity by rheumatologists. Visual loss from lupus retinopathy is viewed as an important index of disease severity [5]. In the pre-steroid era, retinopathy was present in up to half of SLE patients [6]. However, with the advent of steroid and immunosuppressive therapy, the incidence of retinopathy has declined considerably. The prevalence of lupus retinopathy ranges from 3% in an outpatient population with mild to absent disease, to 29% among patients with active disease [7]. The onset of retinopathy may be associated with exacerbation of systemic SLE [8]. The lesions of lupus retinopathy are varied in appearance but most arise from retinal vasculitis.

Retinal Vacular Abnormailities Associated with SLE

1. VASO-Occlusion

A. Microvascular Occlusion

Cotton-wool spots are the classic lesions of SLE retinopathy, represent focal areas of ischemia where there is interruption of axoplasmic flow within the nerve fibers of the retina and are believed to result from occlusion of the small retinal arterioles by infiltrating inflammatory cells. On fluorescein angiography, cotton-wool spots correspond to areas of focal non-perfusion. In contrast to retinal non-perfusion from hypertension and diabetes, the ischemia produced in lupus retinopathy is often not as extensive and is not associated with arterial narrowing [9].

B. Arterial Occlusion

This is a less common form of lupus retinopathy characterized by occlusion of the central retinal artery causing severe retinal ischemia and severe, permanent visual loss [10]; this includes a rapid-onset, painless blurring of vision, a Marcus-Gunn afferent papillary defect, macular ischemia and retinal whitening that results in a 'cherry-red' spot appearance of the fovea [4,9]. Sudden visual loss with central retinal artery occlusion in a young patient should prompt the clinician to include SLE and other collagen disease in the differential diagnosis.

C. Venous Occlusion

SLE is not principally a venous disease, but central retinal vein occlusion has been reported to occur in association with SLE. It may be that an initial arterial occlusion causes secondary venous stasis and engorgement leading to central or branch vein occlusion. Subsequent reperfusion of the arteries, coupled with inflammatory damage to the venous endothelium, may lead to retinal and papillary hemorrhage. Venous occlusion is a rare manifestation of lupus retinopathy but can be a cause of a permanent visual loss [10-11].

2. Vasodisruption

Intraretinal hemorrhages are a frequent finding in SLE retinopathy. Some authors believe that the presence of retinal hemorrhages is a significant finding because it is associated with a greater risk of mortality [12].

A. Ischemic Sequelae

Severe ischemia may result in retinal neovascularization [3,13], the complications of which – vitreous hemorrhage, traction retinal detachment and neovascular glaucoma may be sight threatening.

3. Hypertensive Sequelae

Renal involvement by SLE in general leads to secondary hypertension. When prolonged, the retina may develop hypertensive retinopathy characterized by bilateral retinal arterial narrowing, arteriovenous crossing changes, intraretinal hemorrhages, hard exudate formation and hypertensive papilledema. Occasionally, choroidal infarction may present as foci of underlying choriocapillaries nonperfusion on fluorescein angiography [14].

Similar to diabetic retinopathy, an early lesion in SLE retinopathy may be the retinal capillary microaneurysms. A fluorescein angiographic study of active and inactive SLE patients revealed microaneurysms and/or retinal capillary dilation that leaked fluorescein in 13/50 (24%) consecutive patients. It is not yet clear if these microaneurysms represent the earliest lesions or residual lesions from previous inflammatory episodes [15].

In a study by Lanham et al. [7] the authors concluded that severe retinal vasculitis may occur without systemic illness. This study failed to find an association between retinopathy and cerebral disease [7].Lupus choriodopathy presents as single or multiple areas of serous elevation of the retinal pigment epithelium and sensory retina with associated retinal pigment epithelial mottling. Lupus choriodopathy is highly associated with systemic involvement and is responsive to immunomodulatory therapy.

Vascular lesions in the eye may mirror vascular alterations in the other parts of the body. Thickening of the retinal vessel walls, as well as deposition of fibrinoid material causing vaso-occlusion in the superficial and deep nerve fiber layers has been observed and described in the literature [15-17]. In severe vascular involvement, widespread necrosis of the retina with lymphocytic and plasma cell infiltration may be observed. The similar pathologic lesions of retina and CNS vasculature are well described and may account for the association between retinal and CNS involvement [18-19].

VI. Retinal Vasculitis in other Rheumatic Systemic Autoimmune Diseases

1. Rheumatoid Arthrirtis

The concept of rheumatoid vasculitis started to evolve in the 1960s, when vasculitis with significant clinical manifestations (skin rash, cutaneous ulcerations, gangrene, peripheral neuropathy, and visceral infarction) was described in RA patients [20-22]. Forty years later there is still no universally accepted definition of rheumatoid vasculitis. In practice, rheumatoid vasculitis is considered when clinical manifestations of vasculitis with intraocular inflammation unexplained by conditions such as diabetes, atherosclerosis, infection, drug hypersensitivity, malignancy, or other vasculitides (Wegener's granulomatosis, cryoglobulinemia, polyarteritis nodosa) occur in a patient with an established diagnosis of RA.

Approximately 16% of patients with RV have ophthalmic manifestations [23]; among them, one of the most severe is peripheral ulcerative keratitis (PUK, or "corneal melt"), a condition characterized by inflammation and thinning of the peripheral cornea that may lead to perforation and blindness. Symptoms consist of foreign body sensation with or without eye pain, tearing, photophobia, and reduced visual acuity. In a patient with RA, PUK usually heralds systemic vasculitis and, if left untreated, is associated not only with visual loss, but also with a mortality rate up to 30% [24]. Retinal vasculitis and geographic chorioditis has also been reported to occur in patients with RA [25].

2. Sarcoidosis

Ocular manifestations of the disease have been reported in up to 50% of patients with biopsy-proven disease. Although ocular sarcoidosis tends to initially present as anterior granulomatous uveitis, a wide spectrum of ocular involvement exists. Typical posterior segment findings of sarcoidosis include vitritis with or without inflammatory "snowballs", retinal periphlebitis, preretinal inflammatory nodules and "candle wax drippings" [26,27]. Choroidal lesions have also been reported in ocular sarcoidosis [27,28].

Retinal vasculitis is a characteristic feature of sarcoidosis. It is nearly always a retinal periphlebitis and retinal arteries are only rarely involved in contrast to SLE-RV. The involvement of vessels is discontinuous (in contrast to SLE –RV), and this appears clinically as skip lesions. It may be mild and associated with peripheral retinal and focal vitreal infiltrates indinstiguishable from idiopathic pars planitis (exudates at anterior retina) . RV may be the presenting sign in patients who develop sarcoidosis many years later. In some cases, a more severe periphlebitis develops [29-30]. In the acute stage, this may be accompanied by retinal hemorrhage and edema. With systemic corticosteroid treatment, periphlebitis resolves, but some residual sheathing (longitudal vessel wall exudates that appear like a sheath along vessels) may persist. Yellow perivenous exudates, described as "taches de bougie" (candle-wax drippings) are also sometimes seen, supportive of a clinical diagnosis of sarcoidosis [31].

3. Adamantiades-Behcet's Disease

Adamantiades-Behçet's disease (ABD) is a multisystem vasculitis of unknown etiology, affecting both arteries and veins of all sizes. Ocular involvement occurs in approximately 70% of patients with ABD and is characterized by recurrent, explosive exacerbations of intraocular inflammation most commonly presenting as a posterior uveitis or panuveitis accompanied by an obliterative retinal vasculitis [32,33]. The recurrent exacerbations of severe uveitis can lead to irreversible damage to the retina resulting in significant visual impairment or blindness in 25-50% of affected patients irrespective of immunosuppressive treatment [34]. It has a relapsing-remitting course. Recurrent episodes of intraocular inflammation may eventually lead to blindness. Consequently, aggressive treatment of ocular ABD with systemic corticosteroids alone or in combination with systemic immunomodulatory therapies is recommended at the first onset of posterior segment involvement [35].

Prognosis for eye disease in ABD has improved substantially with the use of conventional immunosuppressive agents such as azathioprine and/or cyclosporine as well interferon (Alpha 2A) and TNF inhibitor. However, despite aggressive treatment with conventional immunosuppressive agents a group of patients still experiences relapses of uveitis. This particular group of

ABD patients with refractory and sight threatening uveitis presents a great challenge to ophthalmologist.

4. Wegener's Granulomatosis

Ocular or orbital involvement of Wegener's granulomatosis (WG) is seen in approximately 29-52% of the patients. [36-38]Approximately 15% of WG patients may present with ocular or orbital disease initially. [38]Although the most common manifestation is orbital granuloma, WG can affect any ocular or periocular tissue. [36,37]In the anterior segment, patients with WG may develop peripheral ulcerative keratitis, corneal granuloma, episcleritis, necrotizing scleritis or uveitis. [39,40]

Retinal involvement is a relatively uncommon ophthalmic manifestation of WG (5-12%), with retinal hemorrhages in the peripheral or posterior retina being the most common finding [41-46]. Both central artery and vein occlusion have been reported [42-44,46]; the exact etiology, however, whether vasculitic, embolic, thrombotic or a retro-orbital process, has not always been clearly defined. Retinal vasculitis, in the form of arteritis or periphlebitis, is a relatively uncommon finding [43,45,46]and may be seen with associated scleritis [45].

5. HLA-B27-Associated Uveitis and Spondyloarthropathies

Uveitis occurring in patients with the HLA-B27 haplotype is a distinct, well recognized clinical entity, characterized by acute, recurrent attacks of inflammation. It usually manifests as a recurrent acute anterior inflammation [47], but according to various studies posterior segment involvement can occur in up to 20% of the patients [48-50], as vitritis, retinal vasculitis, macular edema or papillitis. The presence of the HLA-B27 haplotype in a uveitis patient, either with or without systemic disease, confers added risk for a greater number of complications, compared to patients with idiopathic anterior uveitis; eleven percent of the eyes may eventually be blind, according to data from Power and associates [49]. Rodriguez et al. [51] found posterior segment involvement in 34 eyes of the 29 patients. The most common finding was severe and diffuse vitritis in 93.1% of the patients and papillitis in 24 patients (82.7%). Retinal vasculitis occurred in seven patients (24.1%), and pars plana exudates were present in two patients (6.8%). The study concluded that HLA-

B27-associated uveitis may be related to severe, sight-threatening posterior segment manifestations in some patients; this is an under-recognized phenomenon.

IV. Treatment

The extent of disease, its severity and specific organ involvement are the factors that will determine the type of treatment for patients with RV. The general goals of therapy are to induce remission of the disease, maintain remission and prevent relapses. Most importantly, these goals need to be achieved with minimal morbidity caused by the therapy used or by the disease itself. [52] Patients with ophthalmic manifestations need systemic treatment of the vasculitis in order to achieve control of the ocular inflammation, sparing the excessive use of topical steroids and preventing their complications.

It is important to have assessed the patient for infection with a careful history of eye and physical exams. Laboratory tests, including serology, chest radiograph, and if necessary, vitreous humor analysis, are tailored according to any findings on history and examination.

If infection is identified, appropriate antimicrobial or antiviral therapy is mandatory before attempting immunosuppression. Likewise, identification of any underlying systemic disease is important, not only to help direct therapy for the ocular inflammation but also to control life-threatening complication of autoimmune diseases. Ocular TB, herpetic diseases and lymphoproliferative disorders can mimic retinal vasculitis and in some settings my have systemic symptoms to simulate a rheumatologic condition. Sweets syndrome and Kawasaki syndrome can present with a clinical picture indistinguishable from RV as also can anti- phospholipid syndrome and fibromuscular dysplasia.

Medical Therapy

1. Corticosteroids

These may be administered topically to control anterior uveitis, regionally as subtenon or peribulbar injections for mild unilateral disease, or systemically—orally and also by intravenous pulse therapy. Therapy for RV is more typically systemic and can be initiated with oral corticosteroids that are augmented with immunomodulatory agents similar to those used for rheumatologic conditions.

2. Immunomodulators

To reduce or eliminate the total steroid dose or in cases where RV is poorly controlled, immunomodulators are often required to treat both the ocular inflammation and the systemic manifestations of the disease [53]. Immunomodulators include antimetabolites (methotrexate, azathioprine, calcineurin inhiitors (cyclosporine) and mycophenolate mofetil), alkylating agents (cyclophosphamide, chlorambucil), and biologics (etanercept, infliximab, daclizumab). For patients with poor response to treatment and severe disease, other forms of therapies have been used with some success. Intravenous immunoglobulin (IVIg) therapy has successfully induced remission in patients with active vasculitis, while exchange plasmapheresis has been used to treat severe active diseases with renal failure. [54] Some of the drugs have been favored for certain conditions such as MTX for sarcoid RV, and cyclosporine for macular edema with RV.

3. Intravitreal Anti-vascular Endothelial Growth Factor (VEGF) and Corticosteroids

VEGF is increased in the retina of patients with ocular inflammatory disease or infection. [11] There are accumulating reports on anti-VEGF intravitreal injections for the management of complications of RV [56]. At a recent plenary conference a large series of patients with neovascularization secondary to RV on immunosuppressives demonstrated long term response to periodic bevacizumab (Mansour, Kurup: World Ophthalmology Congress, Berlin. 2010). Intravitreal corticosteroids can help macular edema temporarily until definitive therapy is instituted.

Conclusion

The myriad manifestations(?) of ocular disease in patients with rheumatologic syndromes makes it imperative that a diagnosis of RV is not overlooked. Often, a delay in suspecting RV can be devastating to the patient and the physician, since RV can be rapidly progressive and occlusive. This is especially true in ABD and SLE. The reader is encouraged to review the references or further reading since expansion of many of the concepts described above are beyond the scope of this limited review. Rheumatologists should be aware of the potential of severe visual disability in patients with systemic rheumatologic disease.

References

[1] Gritz DC, Wong IG. Incidence and prevalence of uveitis in Northern California; the Northern California Epidemiology of Uveitis Study. *Ophthalmology* 2004;111:491-500.

[2] Foster CS. Ocular manifestations of the nonrheumatic acquired collagen vascular diseases. In: Smolin G, Thoft RA, eds. T*he Cornea: Scientific Foundations and Clinical Practice.* 2nd ed. Boston: Little, Brown 1987, p.352-357.

[3] Jabs DA, Fine SL, Hochberg MC, et al. Severe retinal vaso-occlusive disease in systemic lupus erythematosus. *Arch Ophthalmol* 1986;104:588.

[4] Wong K, Ai E, Jones JV, Young D. Visual loss as the initial symptom of systemic lupus erythematosus. *Am J Ophthalmol* 1981;92:238.

[5] Committee on Prognosis Studies in SLE: Prognosis Studies in SLE: An activity index (abstract). *Arthritis Rheum* 1986;29:S93.

[6] Baehr G, Klemperer P, Schifrin A. A diffuse disease of the peripheral circulation (usually associated with lupus erythematosus and endocarditis). *Trans Assoc Am Physicians* 1935;50:139.

[7] Lanham JG, Barrie T, Kohner EM, Hughs RV. SLE retinopathy: Evaluation by fluorescein angiography. *Ann Rheum Dis* 1982;41:473

[8] Klinkhoff AV, Beattie CW, Chalmers A. Retinopathy in systemic lupus erythematosus. Relationship to disease activity. *Arthritis Rheum* 1986;29:1152.

[9] Dougal MA, Evans LS, McClellan KR, Robinson J. Central retinal arterial occlusion in systemic lupus erythematosus. *Ann Ophthalmol* 1983;15:38.

[10] Ellis CJ, Hamer DB, Hunt TW, et al. Medical investigation of retinal vascular occlusions. *Br Med J* 1964;2:1093.

[11] Harvey AM, Shulman LE, Tumulty PA, et al. Systemic lupus erythematosus: Review of the literature and clinical analysis of 138 cases. *Medicine* 1954;33:291.

[12] Stafford-Brady FJ, Urowitz MB, Gladman DD, Easterbrook M. Lupus retinopathy: Patterns, associations and prognosis. *Arthritis Rheum* 1988;31:1105.

[13] Kayazawa F, Honda A. Severe retinal vascular lesions in systemic lupus erythematosus. *Ann Ophthalmol* 1981;13:1291.

[14] Carpenter MT, O'Doyle JE, Enzenauer RV, et al. Chorioditis in systemic lupus erythematosus. *Am J Ophthalmol* 1994;117:535-536.

[15] Santos R, Barojas E, Alarcon-Segovia D, Ibanez G. Retinal microangiopathy in systemic lupus erythematosus. *Am J Ophthalmol* 1975;80:249.

[16] Jabs DA, Hanneken AM, Schachat AP, Fine SL. Choriodopathy in systemic lupus erythematosus. *Arch Ophthalmol* 1988;106:230.

[17] Tan EM, Cohen AS, Fries JF, et al. The 1982 revised criteria for the classification of systemic lupus erythematosus. *Arthritis Rheum* 1982;25:1271.

[18] Maumenee AE. Retinal lesions in lupus erythematosus. *Am J Ophthalmol* 1940;23:971.

[19] Graham EM, Spalton DJ, Barnard RO, et al. Cerebral and retinal vascular changes in systemic lupus erythematosus. *Ophthalmology* 1985;92:444-448.

[20] Schmid FR, Cooper NS, Ziff M, McEwan C. Arteritis in rheumatoid arthritis. *Am J Med* 1961;30:56.

[21] Bywaters EGL, Scott JT. The natural history of vascular lesions in rheumatoid arthritis. *J Chronic Dis* 1963;16:905.

[22] Wikinson M, Torrance WN. Clinical background of rheumatoid vascular disease. *Ann Rheum Dis* 1967;26:475.

[23] Scott DG, Bacon PA, Tribe CR. Systemic rheumatoid vasculitis: a clinical and laboratory study of 50 cases. *Medicine (Baltimore)* 1981;60:288-97.

[24] Foster CS, Yee M. Corneoscleral manifestations of Graves' disease, the acquired connective tissue disorders, and systemic vasculitis. *Int Ophthalmol Clin* 1983;23:131-57.

[25] Matsuo T, Masuda I, Matsuo N. Geographic choroiditis and retinal vasculitis in rheumatoid arthritis. *Jpn J Ophthalmol* 1998;42:51-5.

[26] Hunter DG, Foster CS : Ocular manifestations of sarcoidosis. In: Albert DM & Jakobiec FA (eds). Principles and Practice of Ophthalmology. Philadelphia: *WB Saunders* 1994;443–450.

[27] Smith JA, Foster CS. Sarcoidosis and its ocular manifestations. *Int Ophthalmol Clin.* 1996;36:109-25.

[28] Ghabrial R, McCluskey PJ, Wakefield D. Spectrum of sarcoidosis involving the eye and brain. *Aust N Z J Ophthalmol.* 1997;25:221-4.

[29] Spalton D, Sanders M. Fundus changes in histologically confirmed sarcoidosis. *Br J Ophthalmol* 1981;65:348-358.

[30] Bisighini S, Pagluiso L. Retinal vasculitis: A diagnostic dilemma. *Clin Eye Vis Care* 1997;9:71-84.

[31] Graham E, Stanford MR, Sanders MD, et al. A point prevalence study of 150 patients with retinal vasculitis: 1. Diagnostic value of ophthalmologic features. *Br J Ophthalmol* 1989;73:714-721.

[32] Kitaichi N, Miyazaki A, Iwata D, et al. Ocular features of Behçet's disease: An international collaborative study. *Br J Ophthalmol* 2007;91:1579-1582.

[33] Evereklioglu C. Current Concepts in the Etiology and Treatment of Behçet Disease. *Surv Ophthalmol* 2005;50:297-350.

[34] Kötter I, Zierhut M, Eckstein AK, et al. Human recombinant interferon alfa-2a for the treatment of Behçet's disease with sight threatening posterior or panuveitis. *Br J Ophthalmol* 2003;87:423-431.

[35] Jabs DA, Rosenbaum JT, Fosters CS, et al. Guidelines for the Use ofImmunosuppressive Drugs in Patients With Ocular Inflammatory Disorders: Recommendations of an Expert Panel. *Am J Ophthalmol* 2000;130:492-513.

[36] Bullen CL, Liesegang TJ, McDonald TJ, et al. Ocular complications of Wegener's granulomatosis. *Ophthalmology* 1983;90:279-90.

[37] Haynes BF, Fishman ML, Fauci AS, et al. The ocular manifestations of Wegener's granulomatosis. Fifteen years experience and review of the literature. *Am J Med* 1977;63:131-41.

[38] Hoffman GS, Kerr GS, Leavitt RY, et al. Wegener granulomatosis: an analysis of 158 patients. *Ann Intern Med.* 1992;116:488-98.

[39] Kaufman AH, Niles JL, Foster CS. ANCA test in ophthalmic inflammatory disease. *Int Ophthalmol Clin.* 1994;34:215-27.

[40] Power WJ, Rodriguez A, Neves RA, et al. Disease relapse in patients with ocular manifestations of Wegener granulomatosis. *Ophthalmology.* 1995;102:154-60.

[41] Straatsma BR. Ocular manifestation of WG. *Am J Ophthalmol* 1957;144:789.

[42] Haynes BF, Fishman ML, Fauci AS, Wolff SM. The ocular manifestations of Wegener's granlomatosis. Fifteen years experience and review of the literature. *Am J Med* 1977;63:131-141.

[43] Bullen CL, Liesegang TJ, McDonald TJ, DeRemee RA. Ocular complications of WG. *Ophthalmology* 1983;90:279-290.

[44] Pinching AJ, Lockwood CM, Pussell BA, et al. Wegener's granulomatosis: observations on 18 patients with severe renal disease. *Q J Med* 1983;208:435-460.

[45] Cassan SM, Coles DT, Harrison E. The concept of limited forms of Wegener's granulomatosis. *Am J Med* 1970;49:366.

[46] Spalton DJ, Graham EM, Page NGR, Sanders MD. Ocular changes in limited forms of Wegener's granulomatosis. *Br J Ophthalmol* 1981;65:553-563.

[47] Smith RJ. HLA-B27- associated uveitis. *Ophthalmol Clin N Am* 2002;15:297-307

[48] Dodds EM Lowder CY, Meisler DM. Posterior segment inflammation in HLA-B27+ acute anterior uveitis: clinical characteristics. *Ocul Immunol Inflamm* 1999;7:85-92.

[49] Power WJ, Rodriguez A, Pedroza-Seres M, et al. Outcomes in anterior uveitis associated with the HLA-B27 haplotype. *Ophthalmology* 1998;105:1646-1651.

[50] Rodriguez A, Calonge M, Pedrosa-Seres M, et al. Referral patterns of uveitis in a tertiary eye care center. *Arch Ophthalmol* 1996;114:593-9

[51] Rodriguez A, Akova YA, Pedroza-Seres M, Foster CS. Posterior segment ocular manifestations in patients with HLA-B27-associated uveitis. *Ophthalmology* 1994;101:1267-74.

[52] Watts RA, Scott DG, Pusey CD and Lockwood CM. Vasculitis-aims of therapy. An overview. *Rheumatology*. 2000;39:229-237.

[53] Hemady R, Tauber J, Foster CS. Immunosuppressive drugs in immune and inflammatory ocular disease. *Surv Ophthalmol.* 1991;35:369-385.

[54] Perez VL, Chavala SH, Ahmed M, Chu D, et al. Ocular manifestations and concepts of systemic vasculitides. *Surv Ophthalmol* 2004;49:399-418.

[55] Kurup S. Noncorticosteroid Immune Therapy for Ocular Inflammation. In: Tasman W, Jaeger EA, eds. *Duane's Ophthalmology,* Chptr 31. Lippincott Williams & Wilkins, 2008.

[56] Kurup S, Lew J, Byrnes G, et al. Therapeutic efficacy of intravitreal bevacizumab on posterior uveitis complicated by neovascularization. *Acta Ophthalmol.* 2009;87:349-52.

In: Advances in Eye Research. Volume 1 ISBN 978-1-61324-169-1
Editor: W. L. Thomsen, pp. 131-146

Chapter VI

Clinical and Immunopathological Highlights of Non-Infectious Uveitis

Theresa Larson, Nida Sen, Chi-Chao Chan *
Laboratory of Immunology, National Eye Institute, National Institutes of Health, Bethesda, MD, USA

Abstract

Uveitis is a generic term used to describe intraocular inflammation occurring anywhere within the eye. It arises from a diverse group of diseases and is commonly classified based on its location within the eye as anterior, intermediate, posterior, or panuveitis. This review focuses on noninfectious or autoimmune uveitis and its associated immune-pathology. Intraocular inflammation can be acute or chronic. Acute inflammation is marked by infiltration of neutrophils and macrophages while chronic inflammation is marked by infiltration with lymphocytes and macrophages. From an immunopathologic perspective intraocular inflammation can be further studied by the dominating inflammatory cells and their subsets, their inflammatory products including cytokines and immunoglobulins, and the ocular resident cells whose own cell surface markers and adhesion molecules are altered by inflammation. By describing the clinical features of noninfectious uveitis and correlating it with its underlying immunopathology, it will hopefully lead to further clarification of the immunopathogenesis.

Introduction

Uveitis is a descriptive term referring to inflammation of the uvea (iris, ciliary body, and choroid) but is commonly used for inflammation involving any of the intraocular structures (including the vitreous, retina, and choroid). It does not indicate the etiology or pathology, and can be further classified as either autoimmune (noninfectious) or infectious. The current classification scheme used to describe uveitis is based on the International Uveitis Study Group definitions which are also endorsed by the Standardization of Uveitis Nomenclature (SUN) working group. According to the SUN criteria, uveitis is classified based on the anatomic location of the predominating site of inflammation. Uveitis is classified as anterior uveitis if the inflammation involves the iris and ciliary body, intermediate uveitis if the inflammation involves the pars plana and vitreous, posterior uveitis if the inflammation involves the choroid and retina, and finally, panuveitis if the inflammation involves the entire uvea. [1]

Untreated uveitis can lead to serious visual complications and accounts for approximately 10% of visual handicap in the West. It leads to 30,000 new cases of blindness each year at an incidence of 20 – 52 cases per 100,000 person-years and prevalence of 115.3 per 100,000 persons. [2-4] It often affects the working age population with a mean age of onset of 37.2 years old (range 20 – 50 years). [3] It is estimated that 5 – 10% of uveitis cases occur in children less than 16 years of age. [5]

In retrospective studies of uveitis patients, between 35 - 70% displayed some degree of visual impairment or blindness (defined as worse than 20/60 and 20/200). [6-7] In uveitis, complications such as cystoid macular edema (CME) and cataract were frequent, occurring in more than one-half of patients. [6] Prognostic factors predictive of a poor outcome included an anatomical diagnosis of panuveitis, bilateral inflammation, and longer duration of decreased vision. [7]

There are many causes of uveitis both infectious and noninfectious. Infectious etiologies include toxoplasmosis, toxocariasis, syphillis, bartonella, and Lyme disease and commonly encountered noninfectious etiologies can include sarcoidosis, Wegener's granulomatosis, systemic lupus erythematosus or Behcet's disease all of which may have serious systemic implications. Uveitis can also be idiopathic and limited only to the eye as in birdshot retinochoroiditis or serpiginous choroidopathy, entities known as white dot syndromes. Patients presenting with uveitis undergo an extensive diagnostic work up including a history, thorough review of systems, eye exam, laboratory investigations, and imaging based on their pattern of inflammation and systemic symptoms. Despite an extensive workup, 30-50% of patients may still have an idiopathic uveitic diagnosis. [8-11] In this chapter, we will focus on autoimmune or noninfectious uveitis and its associated pathology.

Clinical Features

Anterior uveitis is the most common form of uveitis. Depending on the type of practice, it can account for up to 60 – 90% of all uveitis patients. [10] Anterior uveitis, similar to other forms of uveitis, can be idiopathic and isolated without a systemic disease, associated with systemic autoimmune disease, or infectious. A list of commonly associated diseases includes HLA-B27 associated spondyloarthropathies (although HLAB27 associated anterior uveitis in the absence of spondyloarthropathy also exists), Juvenile Idiopathic Arthritis (JIA), Behcet's disease, sarcoidosis, and syphilis. Glaucomatocyclic crises (Possner-Schlossman Syndrome) and Fuchs heterochromia, previously believed to be idiopathic anterior uveitis syndromes, are now considered viral uveitis syndromes. [12-15] Masquerade syndromes may also present as anterior uveitis. One of the first HLA genetic associations with human disease was HLA-B27 acute anterior uveitis (AAU). [16] It occurs with ocular inflammation either alone or in association with systemic disease. HLA-B27 AAU onset is acute with frequent recurrences and has a typical non-granulomatous appearance. [17] In children, JIA is one of the most common systemic associations. It occurs in children less than 16 years old with arthritis of unknown etiology lasting for at least 6 weeks. Uveitis occurs most commonly in pauciarticular JIA (70%), followed by polyarticular JIA (33%), and is very rare in systemic onset JIA (2%). [18] Most at risk for uveitis are girls with pauciarticular-onset JIA, with a positive antinuclear antibody and negative rheumatoid factor. [19]

Intermediate uveitis accounts for approximately 15% of all cases of uveitis. Most common causes are sarcoidosis, pars planitis syndrome, multiple sclerosis (MS), masquerade syndromes, and infectious causes such as toxoplasmosis, Lyme disease, toxocariasis, syphilis, and tuberculosis. In intermediate uveitis, there is vitritis with and without periphlebitis, snowballs, and snowbanks, a descriptive term referring to inflammatory exudates overlying the ora serrata. Pars planitis is an intermediate uveitis with snowball or snowbank formation without any systemic or infectious association. [1] However, approximately 15% of patients with pars planitis may go on to develop MS. [20] The main vision threatening complication in intermediate uveitis is CME.

Posterior and/or panuveitis comprise approximately 10 – 15% of cases of uveitis. [10] In posterior uveitis there is evidence of retinal inflammation involving a focal choroiditis or retinitis and/or multifocal choroiditis or retinitis. Table 1 shows the multiple causes of posterior or panuveitis. Inflammation in posterior or panuveitis may lead to optic nerve edema, papillitis, or granuloma formation. However, structural complications alone, such as CME or optic nerve edema, are not enough to classify uveitis as posterior in the absence of chorioretinal lesions. [1] The retinal vasculature may show staining, leakage, and capillary dropout on fluorescein angiogram. Inflammation may preferentially involve the veins versus the arteries (such as in Behcet's disease (Figure 1), sarcoidosis, and Eales' disease) and may affect more peripheral versus posterior pole vasculature. Chorioretinal lesions can be described as Dalen-Fuchs nodules (Figure 2A), which we will discuss in further detail as well as by their size and age.

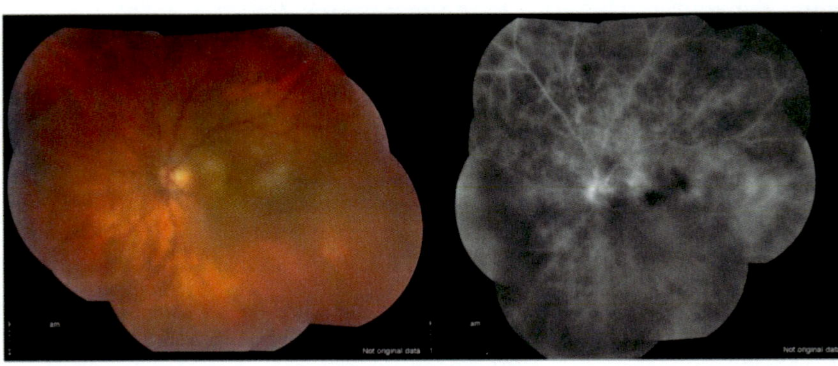

Figure 1. Color fundus photo of Behcet's disease shows (A) areas of active retinitis with inflammation preferentially involving the veins. (B) Fluoroscein angiogram of the same patient demonstrating diffuse vasculitis as well as capillary nonperfusion along the peripheral retina.

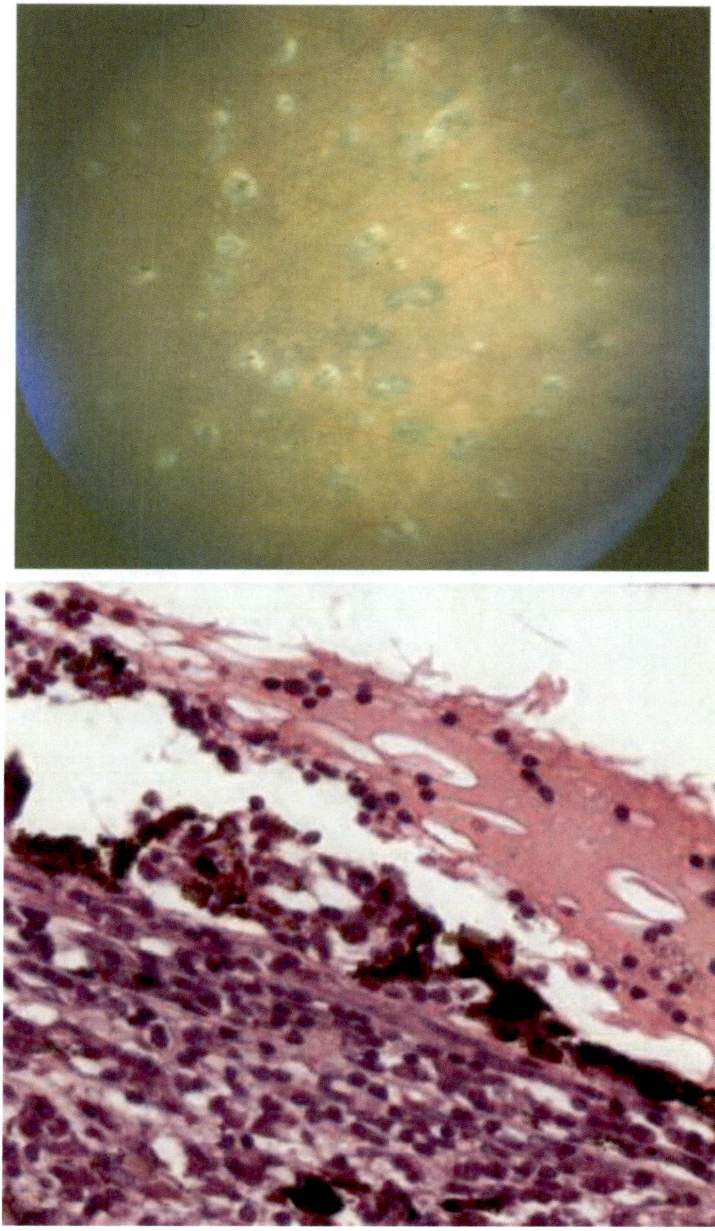

A

B

Figure 2. (A) Punched out chorioretinal lesions demonstrate the typical clinical appearance of Dalen Fuchs nodules. (B) Histopathology of a Dalen Fuchs nodule consisting of a collection of epithelioid-like macrophages between Bruch's membrane and the RPE (hematoxylin-eosin).

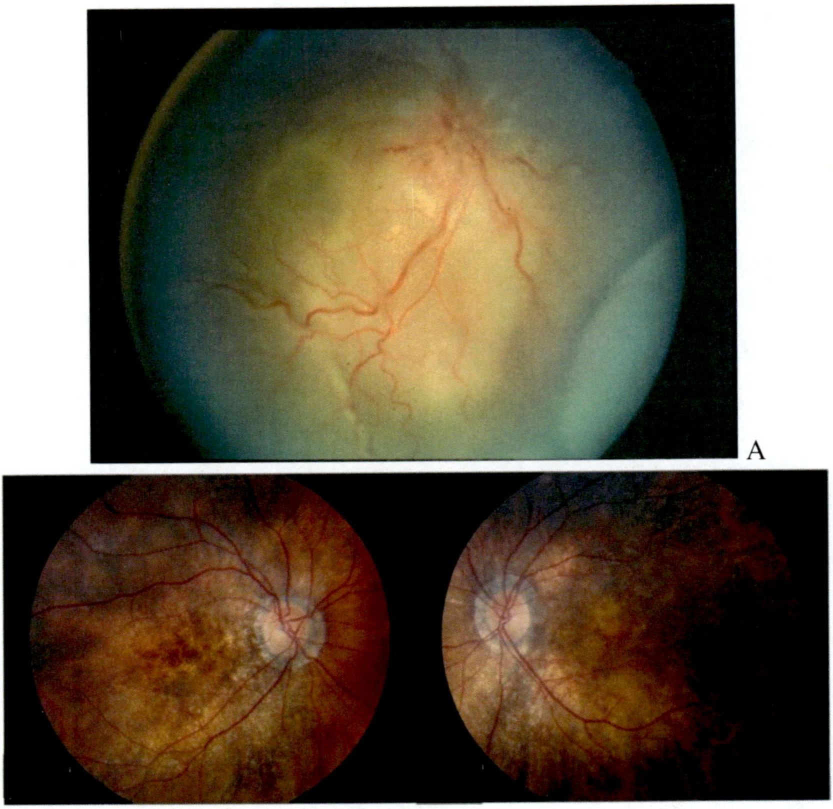

A

B

Figure 3. Fundus photos demonstrate (A) early findings in VKH, optic disc edema, and a large serous retinal detachment. (B) Late findings in VKH include subretinal fibrosis and atrophy.

Systemic diseases commonly associated with uveitis include sarcoidosis, Vogt-Koyanagi-Harada syndrome (VKH, Figure 3A and B), and Behcet's disease. Sarcoidosis is a multisystem granulomatous disease affecting the lungs, skin, eye, lymph nodes, and central nervous system with characteristic noncaseating granulomas. It typically affects young adults and is commonly seen in African Americans and Caucasians of Northern European descent. The etiology is unknown but believed to be immune mediated. Ocular disease is the most common extra-pulmonary presentation occurring in 25 – 50% of patients. [21-23] Anterior uveitis is the most common ocular presentation. Other manifestations in the eye include large granulomatous (mutton-fat) keratic precipitates (Figure 4) and iris nodules in the anterior segment and vitreous cells, snowballs, peripheral perivenous sheathing known as "candle wax drippings," choroidal granulomas, and Dalen-Fuchs nodules in the posterior segment. [24] VKH (Figure 3A and B) is a systemic autoimmune disease affecting the skin, eyes, ears, and meninges. It is common in pigmented ethnic groups with systemic features of vitiligo, alopecia, poliosis, dysacusia, tinnitus, and meningitis. Ocular features include bilateral panuveitis, optic nerve edema, serous retinal detachments, Dalen-Fuchs nodules, and sunset-glow fundus. HLA-DR 4 is commonly associated with VKH in the Japanese. [25] Behcet's disease is a rare multisystem inflammatory disorder with the highest incidence along the ancient Silk Road extending from the Mediterranean basin to Japan. It can affect any organ system but is known for the classical clinical triad of uveitis with oral and genital ulceration. The international study group for Behcet's Disease established diagnostic criteria requiring the presence of oral ulceration with any two of the following: recurrent genital ulcers, ocular inflammation, skin involvement, and positive pathergy test. [26] According to the modified Japanese criteria, four major criteria (skin lesions, oral ulcers, genital ulcers, and ocular inflammation) are required for the diagnosis of the complete type of Behcet's disease followed by incomplete, suspect, and possible types of Behcet's when fewer than four major criteria are met. Ocular disease occurs in explosive, recurrent episodes ranging from an anterior uveitis with a hypopyon to a severe retinitis and retinal vasculitis (Figure 1). [19] The eye can be completely quiet in between episodes. HLA-B51 is commonly associated with Behcet's Disease. [27]

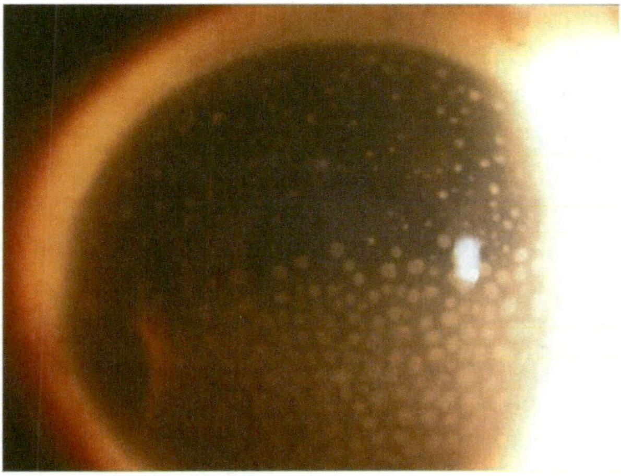

Figure 4. Large mutton fat keratic precipitates in a patient with sarcoidosis.

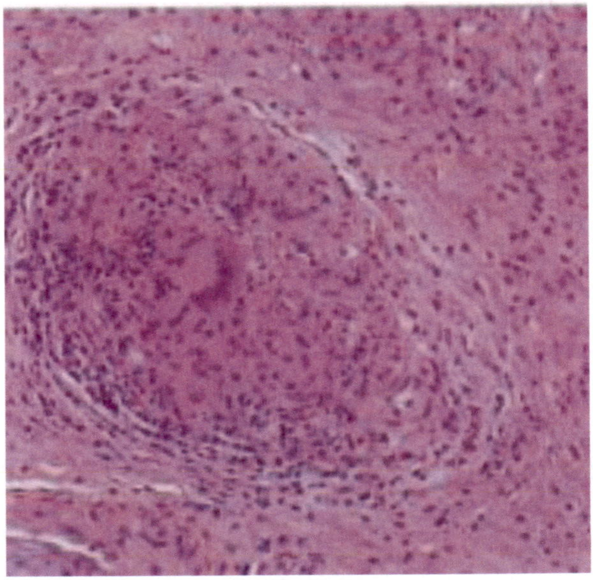

Figure 5. Histopathology of a non-caseating (no necrosis) granuloma with a central multinucleated giant cell and many epithelioid-like macrophages surrounding by lymphocytes. Granulomas are commonly found in diseases such as sarcoidosis, VKH, and sympathetic ophthalmia (hematoxylin-eosin).

Immunopathology

Ocular inflammation, similar to any inflammation, can be examined as acute and chronic inflammation. Acute inflammation occurs within minutes and last hours to several days. It is characterized by fluid exudation and emigration of leukocytes consisting predominantly of neutrophils. Chronic inflammation may follow acute injury or be of insidious onset. It is characterized by lymphocytic and macrophage infiltration, blood vessel proliferation, fibrosis, and tissue necrosis. Subacute inflammation is a transition between acute and chronic and can reflect characteristics from both. Chronic inflammation is further described as granulomatous versus nongranulomatous. A granuloma describes an aggregate consisting of mainly macrophages, some of them may look like epithelioid cells and some may fuse to form multinucleated giant cells (Figure 5). [28] A noncaseating granuloma exhibits histologically intact cells and a caseating granuloma exhibits necrotic centers, such as seen in tuberculosis granulomas.

Table 1. Causes of Posterior And/Or Panuveitis

Focal choroiditis/retinitis:
Toxocariasis
Tuberculosis
Nocardiosis
Masquerade syndrome
Multifocal Choroiditis:
Sympathetic Ophthalmia
Vogt Koyanagi Harada
Sarcoidosis
Serpiginous
Birdshot Choroidopathy
Wegener's
Systemic lupus erythematosis
Histoplasmosis/TB
Masquerade syndrome
Syphilis
Herpes simplex virus
Cytomegalovirus
Sarcoidosis
Masquerade syndromes
Candidiasis
Meningococcus
Panuveitis
Syphilis
Sarcoidosis
Vogt Koyanagi Harada
Behcet's disease
Sympathetic Ophthalmia
Infectious endophthalmitis (bacterial and fungal etiologies)

Intraocular inflammation can be further described by the inflammatory cellular subtypes, inflammatory products, and ocular resident cells involved in uveitic inflammation. The different subsets of inflammatory cells include T and B lymphocytes, macrophages, and granulocytes (or neutrophils). Lymphocytes are further classified by cell surface markers into two broad categories of T lymphocytes (CD3), which are thymus derived and B lymphocytes (CD19) which are bone marrow derived. Multiple subsets of T cells have been described including T helper cells (CD4+, Th), T suppressor/cytotoxic cells (CD8) and many others (*Th1, Th2, Th3, Th17, CTL,* T_M, T_{reg}). [29] Once activated, CD4+ T cells are further subdivided into Th1 and Th2 cells based on their cytokine profile. A third subset has recently been discovered, the IL-17-producing effector T helper cells, Th17. Uveitis is believed to be mainly Th1 and Th17 mediated. [30]

T lymphocytic infiltration is the hallmark of chronic inflammation seen in many uveitic diseases (see Table 2). Pathologically, this was demonstrated in a series of iridectomy specimens from patients with quiescent chronic uveitis which included anterior, intermediate, posterior, and panuveitis. In 9 of 16 iridectomy specimens there was predominant T lymphocytic infiltration (interleukin-2 receptor-negative T helper and suppressor cells) compared to none of the control specimens. Class II antigens were also detected in the iris stroma in all uveitis patients and only six of the eleven control patients. [31] In an enucleated eye with pars planitis, there was T lymphocyte infiltration in the overlying snow bank in the pars plana. [32] In posterior uveitis such as inflammatory Coats disease characterized by massive retinal exudation and vascular anomalies, an enucleated eye revealed perivascular lymphocytic infiltration with CD4+ T cells. [33]

Table 2. Predominant T lymphocytic Infiltration in Non-Infectious Uveitis

Anterior Uveitis, idiopathic:	non-granulomatous inflammation
Behcet's Disease:	non-granulomatous inflammation (majority)
Pars Planitis:	non-granulomatous inflammation
Retinal Vasculitis:	non-granulomatous inflammation (majority)
Sarcoidosis:	non-necrotizing granulomatous inflammation
Scleritis:	granulomatous and non-granulomatous inflammation
Sympathetic Ophthalmia:	non-necrotizing granulomatous inflammation
Vogt-Koyanagi-Harada's Syndrome:	granulomatous and non-granulomatous inflammation
Multifocoal Choroiditis*:	non-granulomatous inflammation
Subretinal Fibrosis with Uveitis*:	non-granulomatous inflammation

* Denotes uveitic diseases with predominantly B cell infiltration.

T lymphocytic infiltration is also seen sympathetic ophthalmia (SO), a rare bilateral granulomatous panuveitis which occurs after surgical or accidental trauma to one eye, the exciting eye, followed by the development of uveitis in the uninjured eye, the sympathizing eye. Part of the histopathology is the presence of Dalen-Fuchs nodules, which are collections of epithelioid macrophages, lymphocytes, and retinal pigment epithelial cells on the inner surface of Bruch's membrane (Figure 2B). In Dalen- Fuchs nodules from an enucleated eye with SO, there were T cells (CD3+) and macrophages. Furthermore, there was a predominant Th1 response over Th2 response from positive interleukin-2 (IL-2) mRNA and negative IL-4 mRNA staining in infiltrating lymphocytes. [29]

Ocular sarcoidosis similarly shows infiltrating macrophages and lymphocytes. Histopathology of an enucleated eye with sarcoidosis revealed an anterior chamber filled with granulomas. The non-caseating granulomas were composed of pale and vacuolated epitheliod cells infiltrated by macrophages as well as CD4+ T-cells. [34]

Fewer uveitic diseases show predominantly B cell infiltration. A chorioretinal biopsy from subretinal fibrosis and uveitis demonstrated a relative increase in B cells and plasma cells. [35] Although VKH and sympathetic ophthalmia have an increase in T cells in earlier stages of the disease, end stage uveitis in these conditions may show a predominance of B cells. [36-37]

The ocular resident cells consist of many different ocular cells which include vascular endothelial cells, pigmented epithelial cells, corneal endothelial cells, fibroblasts, melanocytes, and Muller cells. Their primary role is not immunologic; however, they express antigens involved the inflammatory process. They can alter their surface markers of MHC class I and II antigens and adhesion molecules before inflammatory cells infiltrate the eye. [29] Both the antigen-peptide and MHC complexes are necessary for Th-cell activation. [38] *In vitro* human retinal pigment epithelial (RPE) cells when treated with interferon-γ express MHC class II molecules (HLA-DR) which is an activation marker, and can function as antigen presenting cells. [39-40] In humans, eye sections demonstrated HLA-DR antigens expressed on RPE in uveitic eyes but not on RPE from normal eyes. [41]

Cell adhesion molecules are cell surface glycoproteins that promote migration of leucocytes to areas of inflammation. In the eye, they are expressed on ocular cells with their counter-receptors or ligands on leucocytes. A particular cell adhesion molecule, intercellular adhesion molecule-1 (ICAM-1/CD54) can be expressed on cornea and RPE and when associated with lymphocytes function-associated antigen (LFA-1/CD11a), an integrin, it can participate in lymphocyte migration. [42-43] Evidence supporting their role in uveitis comes from histopathology which showed ICAM-1 expressed in the RPE and LFA-1 along retinal vessels in eyes of patients with posterior uveitis but not normal control eyes. [44]

Apoptosis is important to maintaining the immune privilege of the eye, dysfunction of which may lead to autoimmunity. It is mediated by Fas (CD95) and Fas ligand (FasL). When they bind, the target cell undergoes apoptosis or programmed cell death. In an immune response, it has the potential to eliminate autoreactive and activated T cells. [45] DNA fragmentation, assessed using the TUNEL technique (terminal deoxynucleotidyl transferase-mediated biotin-deoxyuridine triphosphate nick-end labeling), labels the particular cell undergoing apoptosis. In normal eyes Fas and FasL were constituvely expressed predominantly in the retina with very little expression in the choroid; however, in uveitic eyes, there was increased expression in the retina, chorioretinal scars, and chorioretinal granulomas. Taken together, this may indicate dysregulation of Fas and FasL in ocular inflammation. [46]

Other effects on ocular resident cells include upregulation of growth factors in certain disease states. Vascular endothelial growth factor (VEGF), an angiogenic and vasopermeability factor, is induced in retinal ischemia and implicated in age related macular degeneration, retinal vascular occlusions, and diabetic retinopathy. [47-48] In Eale's disease, a primary idiopathic retinal vasculitis and vaso-occlusive disease inducing ischemia and secondary neovascularization; there was intense expression of VEGF and enhanced expression of VEGF mRNA in pre-retinal neovascular membranes. [49] VEGF was also increased in the aqueous of uveitic patients with CME compared to those without CME. [50]

Conclusion

Uveitis refers to a diverse set of diseases, which seem to share common immune mechanisms. They are predominantly T cell mediated diseases with a Th1 and Th17 response. Ocular resident cells are capable of becoming immunologically activated as evidenced by expression HLA DR and cellular adhesion molecules as well as affected by particular growth factors such as VEGF. Apoptotic pathways contribute to the maintenance of the immune environment. All of these pathways contribute to presentation of antigen, activation of Th cells, and consequent recruitment of leukocytes and resultant inflammation. Further understanding of the immune mechanisms and pathological processes will hopefully lead to a better understanding of the multiple manifestations of disease both within the eye and systemically.

References

[1] Jabs DA, Nussenblatt RB, Rosenbaum JT. Standardization of uveitis nomenclature for reporting clinical data. Results of the First International Workshop. *Am J Ophthalmol.* Sep 2005;140(3):509-516.

[2] Nussenblatt RB. The natural history of uveitis. *Int Ophthalmol.* Oct 1990;14(5-6):303-308.

[3] Darrell RW, Wagener HP, Kurland LT. Epidemiology of uveitis. Incidence and prevalence in a small urban community. *Arch Ophthalmol.* Oct 1962;68:502-514.

[4] Gritz DC, Wong IG. Incidence and prevalence of uveitis in Northern California; the Northern California Epidemiology of Uveitis Study. *Ophthalmology.* Mar 2004;111(3):491-500; discussion 500.

[5] Zierhut M, Michels H, Stubiger N, Besch D, Deuter C, Heiligenhaus A. Uveitis in children. *Int Ophthalmol Clin.* Spring 2005;45(2):135-156.

[6] Rothova A, Suttorp-van Schulten MS, Frits Treffers W, Kijlstra A. Causes and frequency of blindness in patients with intraocular inflammatory disease. *Br J Ophthalmol.* Apr 1996;80(4):332-336.

[7] Durrani OM, Tehrani NN, Marr JE, Moradi P, Stavrou P, Murray PI. Degree, duration, and causes of visual loss in uveitis. *Br J Ophthalmol.* Sep 2004;88(9):1159-1162.

[8] Chatzistefanou K, Markomichelakis NN, Christen W, Soheilian M, Foster CS. Characteristics of uveitis presenting for the first time in the elderly. *Ophthalmology.* Feb 1998;105(2):347-352.

[9] Henderly DE, Genstler AJ, Smith RE, Rao NA. Changing patterns of uveitis. *Am J Ophthalmol.* Feb 15 1987;103(2):131-136.

[10] McCannel CA, Holland GN, Helm CJ, Cornell PJ, Winston JV, Rimmer TG. Causes of uveitis in the general practice of ophthalmology. UCLA Community-Based Uveitis Study Group. *Am J Ophthalmol.* Jan 1996;121(1):35-46.

[11] Smith JA, Mackensen F, Sen HN, et al. Epidemiology and course of disease in childhood uveitis. *Ophthalmology.* Aug 2009;116(8):1544-1551, 1551 e1541.

[12] Ruokonen PC, Metzner S, Ucer A, Torun N, Hofmann J, Pleyer U. Intraocular antibody synthesis against rubella virus and other microorganisms in Fuchs' heterochromic cyclitis. *Graefes Arch Clin Exp Ophthalmol.* Apr 2010;248(4):565-571.

[13] Suzuki J, Goto H, Komase K, et al. Rubella virus as a possible etiological agent of Fuchs heterochromic iridocyclitis. *Graefes Arch Clin Exp Ophthalmol.* Oct 2010;248(10):1487-1491.

[14] Chee SP, Jap A. Presumed fuchs heterochromic iridocyclitis and Posner-Schlossman syndrome: comparison of cytomegalovirus-positive and negative eyes. *Am J Ophthalmol.* Dec 2008;146(6):883-889 e881.

[15] Chee SP, Bacsal K, Jap A, Se-Thoe SY, Cheng CL, Tan BH. Clinical features of cytomegalovirus anterior uveitis in immunocompetent patients. *Am J Ophthalmol.* May 2008;145(5):834-840.

[16] Brewerton DA, Caffrey M, Nicholls A, Walters D, James DC. Letter: Acute anterior uveitis and HL-A 27. *Lancet.* Mar 16 1974;1(7855):464.

[17] Chang JH, McCluskey PJ, Wakefield D. Acute anterior uveitis and HLA-B27. *Surv Ophthalmol.* Jul-Aug 2005;50(4):364-388.

[18] Sauberan DP. Pediatric uveitis. *Int Ophthalmol Clin.* Fall 2010;50(4):73-85.

[19] Nussenblatt RW, SM. *Uveitis: Fundamentals and Clinical Practice.* Third ed. Philadelphia: Elsevier; 2004.

[20] Raja SC, Jabs DA, Dunn JP, et al. Pars planitis: clinical features and class II HLA associations. *Ophthalmology.* Mar 1999;106(3):594-599.

[21] James DG, Neville E, Langley DA. Ocular sarcoidosis. *Trans Ophthalmol Soc U K.* Apr 1976;96(1):133-139.

[22] Obenauf CD, Shaw HE, Sydnor CF, Klintworth GK. Sarcoidosis and its ophthalmic manifestations. *Am J Ophthalmol.* Nov 1978;86(5):648-655.

[23] Jabs DA, Johns CJ. Ocular involvement in chronic sarcoidosis. *Am J Ophthalmol.* Sep 15 1986;102(3):297-301.

[24] Herbort CP, Rao NA, Mochizuki M. International criteria for the diagnosis of ocular sarcoidosis: results of the first International Workshop On Ocular Sarcoidosis (IWOS). *Ocul Immunol Inflamm.* May-Jun 2009;17(3):160-169.

[25] Shindo Y, Ohno S, Yamamoto T, Nakamura S, Inoko H. Complete association of the HLA-DRB1*04 and -DQB1*04 alleles with Vogt-Koyanagi-Harada's disease. *Hum Immunol.* Mar 1994;39(3):169-176.

[26] Criteria for diagnosis of Behcet's disease. International Study Group for Behcet's Disease. *Lancet.* May 5 1990;335(8697):1078-1080.

[27] Du L, Kijlstra A, Yang P. Immune response genes in uveitis. *Ocul Immunol Inflamm.* Jul-Aug 2009;17(4):249-256.

[28] Robbins S, Kumar V, Cotran, RS. *Robbins and Cotran pathologic basis of disease.* 8th ed. ed. Philadephia: Saunders/Elsevier; 2010.

[29] Chan CC, Li Q. Immunopathology of uveitis. *Br J Ophthalmol.* Jan 1998;82(1):91-96.

[30] Caspi RR. A look at autoimmunity and inflammation in the eye. *J Clin Invest.* Sep 1 2010;120(9):3073-3083.

[31] Stevens G, Jr., Chan CC, Wetzig RP, Nussenblatt RB, Palestine AG. Iris lymphocytic infiltration in patients with clinically quiescent uveitis. *Am J Ophthalmol.* Nov 15 1987;104(5):508-515.

[32] Wetzig RP, Chan CC, Nussenblatt RB, Palestine AG, Mazur DO, Mittal KK. Clinical and immunopathological studies of pars planitis in a family. *Br J Ophthalmol.* Jan 1988;72(1):5-10.

[33] Lim WK, Nussenblatt RB, Chan CC. Immunopathologic features of inflammatory coats disease. *Arch Ophthalmol.* Feb 2005;123(2):279-281.

[34] Chan CC, Wetzig RP, Palestine AG, Kuwabara T, Nusenblatt RB. Immunohistopathology of ocular sarcoidosis. Report of a case and discussion of immunopathogenesis. *Arch Ophthalmol.* Oct 1987;105(10):1398-1402.

[35] Palestine AG, Nussenblatt RB, Chan CC, Hooks JJ, Friedman L, Kuwabara T. Histopathology of the subretinal fibrosis and uveitis syndrome. *Ophthalmology.* Jun 1985;92(6):838-844.

[36] Shah DN PM, Burnier MN, Jr, McLean IW, Nussenblatt RB, Chan C-C. Inflammatory cellular kinetics in sympathetic ophthalmia. A study of 29 traumatized (exciting) eyes. *Ocular Immunology and Inflammation.* 1993;1(3):8.

[37] Chan CC, Palestine AG, Kuwabara T, Nussenblatt RB. Immunopathologic study of Vogt-Koyanagi-Harada syndrome. *Am J Ophthalmol.* Jun 15 1988;105(6):607-611.

[38] Dong C, Flavell RA. Th1 and Th2 cells. *Curr Opin Hematol.* Jan 2001;8(1):47-51.

[39] Osusky R, Dorio RJ, Arora YK, Ryan SJ, Walker SM. MHC class II positive retinal pigment epithelial (RPE) cells can function as antigen-presenting cells for microbial superantigen. *Ocul Immunol Inflamm.* Mar 1997;5(1):43-50.

[40] Liversidge JM, Sewell HF, Forrester JV. Human retinal pigment epithelial cells differentially express MHC class II (HLA, DP, DR and DQ) antigens in response to in vitro stimulation with lymphokine or purified IFN-gamma. *Clin Exp Immunol.* Sep 1988;73(3):489-494.

[41] Chan CC, Detrick B, Nussenblatt RB, Palestine AG, Fujikawa LS, Hooks JJ. HLA-DR antigens on retinal pigment epithelial cells from patients with uveitis. *Arch Ophthalmol.* May 1986;104(5):725-729.

[42] Elner VM, Elner SG, Pavilack MA, Todd RF, 3rd, Yue BY, Huber AR. Intercellular adhesion molecule-1 in human corneal endothelium. Modulation and function. *Am J Pathol.* Mar 1991;138(3):525-536.

[43] Forrester JV, Liversidge J, Dua HS. Regulation of the local immune response by retinal cells. *Curr Eye Res.* 1990;9 Suppl:183-191.

[44] Whitcup SM, Chan CC, Li Q, Nussenblatt RB. Expression of cell adhesion molecules in posterior uveitis. *Arch Ophthalmol.* May 1992;110(5):662-666.

[45] Lynch DH, Ramsdell F, Alderson MR. Fas and FasL in the homeostatic regulation of immune responses. *Immunol Today.* Dec 1995;16(12):569-574.

[46] Chan CC, Matteson DM, Li Q, Whitcup SM, Nussenblatt RB. Apoptosis in patients with posterior uveitis. *Arch Ophthalmol.* Dec 1997;115(12):1559-1567.

[47] Witmer AN, Vrensen GF, Van Noorden CJ, Schlingemann RO. Vascular endothelial growth factors and angiogenesis in eye disease. *Prog Retin Eye Res.* Jan 2003;22(1):1-29.

[48] Aiello LP, Avery RL, Arrigg PG, et al. Vascular endothelial growth factor in ocular fluid of patients with diabetic retinopathy and other retinal disorders. *N Engl J Med.* Dec 1 1994;331(22):1480-1487.

[49] Perentes Y, Chan CC, Bovey E, Uffer S, Herbort CP. Massive vascular endothelium growth factor (VEGF) expression in Eales' disease. *Klin Monbl Augenheilkd.* Apr 2002;219(4):311-314.

[50] Fine HF, Baffi J, Reed GF, Csaky KG, Nussenblatt RB. Aqueous humor and plasma vascular endothelial growth factor in uveitis-associated cystoid macular edema. *Am J Ophthalmol.* Nov 2001;132(5):794-796.

In: Advances in Eye Research. Volume 1
Editor: W. L. Thomsen, pp. 147-158
ISBN 978-1-61324-169-1

Chapter VII

Vogt-Koyanagi-Harada Disease

Jozélio Freire de Carvalho[1,*], Alexandre Wagner de Souza[2], Joyce Hisae Yamamoto[3] and Simone Appenzeller[4]

[1]Rheumatology Division, Hospital das Clínicas da Faculdade de Medicina da Universidade de São Paulo, São Paulo, SP, Brazil

[2]Rheumatology Division, Faculdade de Medicina da Universidade Federal de São Paulo, São Paulo, SP, Brazil

[3]Ophthalmology Department, Hospital das Clínicas da Faculdade de Medicina da Universidade de São Paulo, São Paulo, SP, Brazil

[4]Rheumatology Division, Hospital das Clínicas da Faculdade de Medicina da Universidade de Campinas, Campinas, Brazil

Abstract

The term panuveitis is reserved for diseases that involve all segments of the uveal tract, including the retina and vitreous body. It is usually

---

* Corresponding author: Jozélio F. Carvalho MD, PhD. Disciplina de Reumatologia, Faculdade de Medicina da USP; Av. Dr. Arnaldo, 455, 3 andar, sala 3133; São Paulo – SP, Brasil, 01246-903; Telephone: 5511-30617492; Fax: 5511-30617490. E-mail: jotafc@gmail.com

Carvalho JF received grants from Federico Foundation and CNPq (300665/2009-1); Apenzeller S received grants from CNPq (2009/06049-6) and FAPESP (2008/02917-0).

associated with severe sight-threatening inflammatory response. The common causes of panuveitis in our population are tuberculosis, syphilis, Vogt-Koyanagi-Harada disease, sympathetic ophthalmia, Behçet's disease and sarcoidosis. Vogt-Koyanagi-Harada disease (VKH) is a multisystem autoimmune disorder affecting pigmented tissues such as the eye, auditory, integumentary and central nervous systems. Patients are typically females between 20 to 50 years old with no previous history of penetrating ocular trauma. Despite the increasing reports published about the clinical features of VKHdisease in various ethnic populations, the etiology of VKH disease is still not completely known. Clinical, laboratorial, experimental data corroborate to the autoimmune nature of VKH disease in a genetically susceptible individual. A stepwise approach is essential while evaluating these patients to be able to identify and treat the disease timely and adequately. Ancillary tests can be appropriately applied once the clinical diagnosis is made. Treatment is based on initial high-dose oral corticosteroids with a low tapering during a minimum period of 6 months. Systemic immunomodulatory agents such as cyclosporine may be used in refractory or corticosteroid non-tolerant patients. Visual prognosis is usually good under a prompt diagnosis and adequate treatment. The aim of this paper is to review the latest research results on VKH disease in order to help to understand better this potentially blinding disease and to improve treatment.

Keywords: uveitis, Vogt-Koyanagi-Harada, diagnostic criteria

1. Introduction

Vogt-Koyanagi-Harada (VKH) disease is a multisystem granulomatous autoimmune disease affecting pigmented tissues of the eye, the central nervous system, internal ear and skin. Patients with bilateral uveitis associated with poliosis, vitiligo, alopecia and dysacusia were first described by Vogt in 1906 and then by Koyanagi in 1929 [1, 2]. In 1926, Harada described a case of uveitis with exudative retinal detachment associated with pleocytosis of the cerebral spinal fluid [3]. VKH disease is a relatively rare systemic disorder with an immunologic etiology in which an autoimmune reaction is directed against melanocyte-containing organs in a genetically susceptible individual, causing bilateral granulomatous panuveitis with choroiditis and exudative retinal detachment. Systemic manifestations include skin, auditory, and central nervous system abnormalities, which may be present to varying extents.

2. Epidemiology

Pigmented races are more commonly affected and VKH disease is rarely observed in Caucasian. Surprisingly, is not described in sub-Saharan African descents [4]. Women are affected more frequently than men and there is a clear predominance in the third to fourth decade of life, although children as young as 4 year-old have been affected. VKH disease is more prevalent in Japan, accounting for 10.1% of all uveitis compared to 1-4% in the US [5] or 2.5% in Brazil [6]. Darkly pigmented races tend to be affected more commonly than non-pigmented races, and the disorder is more commonly seen in Far East Asians, in particular in Japanese, Hispanics, American Indians, and subcontinent Asian Indians. [7].

3. Pathogenesis

Although the etiology of VKH disease remains unknown, several evidences corroborate to the autoimmunity against melanocytes triggered by an unknown factor in a genetically susceptible individual. The prodromic manifestations point to a viral trigger such as family of herpes virus (Epstein-Barr virus, cytomegalovirus). Histopathological findings as well as *in vitro* experiments and animal models reinforce the importance of the CD4+ T lymphocytes in the disease pathogenesis [8]. Several melanocyte derived antigens are being analyzed as the target protein of the disease, especially tyrosinase and tyrosinase related proteins [9]. Since VKH disease has a concentration in some ethnic groups in the world, a genetic background has been suggested. In fact, HLA-DRB1*0405 has been associated with 90% of Asian patients with VKH disease [10] as well as in patients from other countries [11]. Autoimmunity to retinal antigens has also been found in patients with VKH disease [12].

4. Clinical Manifestations

VKH disease has four distinctive phases: prodromal, uveitic, convalescent, and chronic/recurrent. Extra-ocular manifestations are characteristically observed in prodromal, convalescent and chronic phases [7].

The prodromal phase is characterized by generalized symptoms of fever, nausea, and headache which last for three to five days. Subsequently, the uveitic phase starts, with ocular symptoms including photophobia, blurred vision and ocular pain. On examination of the eyes a bilateral, granulomatous anterior uveitis with mutton fat keratic precipitates and iris nodules are observed. In addition, a diffuse choroiditis associated with exudative retinal detachment and optic disc hyperemia are observed. Swelling of the ciliary body may displace the lens-iris diaphragm forward with consequent shallowing of the anterior chamber, angle narrowing and an acute increase in intraocular pressure.

In the convalescent phase, as a result of appropriate treatment, the choroiditis gradually subsides as well as the exudative retinal detachment. In this phase, it is observed the typical "sunset glow" fundus (orange-red fundus appearance), multiple scattered, discrete, depigmented lesions in the mid periphery of the fundus and retinal pigment epithelial migration, all denoting the profound melanocyte and pigmented tissue aggression. Sugiura sign is the depigmentation of limbus mainly reported by Japanese authors. In this phase, cutaneous depigmentation may be observed.

Recurrence or chronicity of the uveitis may occur in 17 to 73% of the patients. The recurrence is usually anterior, nevertheless signs of disease activity in the posterior pole of the eye have been recently reported, suggesting relentless melanocyte aggression [13]. In the convalescent and chronic phases ocular complications such as glaucoma, cataract, choroidal neovascular membrane and retinal/choroidal fibrosis, may be observed. These long-term ocular complications may lead to final low visual acuity.

Extra-ocular manifestations: Nonspecific signs such as fever and nausea in the prodromal phase can occur. The auditory system may be involved by dysacousia, tinnitus, high-frequency hearing loss, and vertigo. In the same manner, the central nervous system can be affected by headache, meningismus, and pleocytosis in the cerebral spine fluid that precede the ocular involvement by one to two weeks. Infrequently, focal neurological signs can develop such as cranial nerve palsies and optic neuritis. Diffuse manifestations such as aphasia, personality changes, loss of consciousness, and seizures characterizing encephalitis can occur. Cutaneous manifestations, commonly observed in the convalescent and chronic phases, are vitiligo of the hands, shoulders, breast, back and face, poliosis, or whitening of a patch of hair, eyebrows or eyelashes and alopecia.

Table 1. American Uveitis Society criteria for diagnosis of VKH disease

No history of trauma or surgery and one finding from at least three of the following four groups:

1. Bilateral chronic iridocyclitis
2. Posterior uveitis: exudative retinal detachment, formed fruste of retinal detachment (disc hyperemia or edema, subretinal macular edema), and "sunset glow" fundus
3. Neurological signs: tinnitus, meningismus, cranial nerve or central nervous system problem, cerebrospinal fluid pleocytosis
4. Cutaneous signs: alopecia, poliosis, or vitiligo

VKH disease is known to have varied manifestations in different ethnic groups. For instance, in Japanese patients, dysacusia occurs in 70–80%, poliosis or alopecia in 60%, and vitiligo in 25%; however, in USA, dysacusia was noted in 8%, poliosis in 25%, and alopecia in 8% of patients [6, 11, 12, 14]. Since the clinical features of VKH vary depending upon the stage of the disease, patients rarely have all of these features during the initial presentation.

Other conditions observed in patients with VKH disease keratoconjunctivitis *sicca* syndrome with a few cases fulfilling diagnostic criteria for Sjögren syndrome and a frequency of 10% anti-Ro/SS-A reactivity has been described in VKH [15]; Guillain-Barré syndrome and glucose intolerance were also reported .

5. Pathological Features

Classical histopathologic findings in the acute phase are a diffuse granulomatous bilateral uveitis. The choroid is remarkably thickened and infiltrated with lymphocytes, machophages, epithelioid cells and giant cells. Another characteristic finding is the Dalen-Fuchs nodules that consisted of macrophages, epithelioid cells, lymphocytes and altered retinal pigment epitethelium cells localized between the Bruch membrane and retinal pigment epithelium. In the convalescent and chronic phases of the disease, disappearance of melanocytes of choroid is described.

Table 2. Sugiura´s diagnostic criteria for VKH disease

1. Acute bilateral uveitis with simultaneous involvement of both eyes. Symptoms may not be noted for 1-10 days in the second eye. 2. Circumscribed retinal edema most markedly at the posterior pole. Fluorescent angiography reveals characteristic leakage of dye through the retinal pigment epithelium into the sub retinal spaces. 3. Pleocytosis of the cerebrospinal fluid is noted in the early stages of the disease. Dysacousia, vertigo, and scalp sensitivity when touching the hair are of value in early diagnosis, if present. Floating cells in the anterior chamber, granulomatous keratic precipitates, and iris nodules are important signs that may be absent in early stages. Hair loss and depigmentation of the eye, skin, and hair are also important signs in the convalescent stage. Depigmentation of the corneal limbus appears earliest (Sigiura´s sign), roughly 1 month after onset, and is also of value for confirming the early diagnosis if present.

Criteria 1, 2 and 3 are major symptoms. Criteria 1 or 2, and 3 are required to diagnose VKH disease. Minor symptoms are noted below the major symptoms and are helpful in diagnosis, if present.

6. Complementary Exams

The diagnosis of VKH disease is basically clinical, nevertheless in atypical cases complementary exams may be helpful. Most of cases are incomplete or probable, so clinical investigations such as fluorescein angiography, lumbar puncture, ultrasound, indocyanine angiography, and optical coherence tomography (OCT) are found useful in substantiating the diagnosis. Transitory pleocytosis is observed in 72% with predominance of lymphomonocytes within the first three weeks after disease onset. Ulltrasonography of the eye reveals low to medium reflective diffuse thickening of choroid with localized and extensive retinal exudative detachment, differentiating VKH from higher reflectivity of idiopathic uveal effusion and metastatic carcinoma. Fluorescein angiography in the acute phase of the disease shows tipically multiple hyperfluorescent pinpoints, corresponding to choroiditis lesions, which coalesce into larger areas corresponding to the retinal exudative detachment.

Table 3. Revised diagnostic criteria for VKH disease

1. No history of penetrating ocular trauma
2. No evidence of other ocular or systemic disease
3. Bilateral ocular disease – either a or b:
   a. Early manifestations
   i. Diffuse choroiditis manifested as either;
      1. Focal areas of sub retinal fluid or
      2. Bullous serous retinal detachment
   ii. If equivocal fundus findings then both of below
      1. Fluorescent angiography showing focal delayed choroidal perfusion, pinpoint leakage, pooling within subretinal fluid, and optic nerve staining
      2. Ultrasound showing diffuse choroidal thickening without posterior scleritis
   b. Late manifestations
   i. History suggestive of above, and both ii and iii or multiple from iii
   ii. Ocular depigmentation
      1. Sunset glow fundus, or
      2. Sugiura´s sign
   iii. Other ocular signs
      1. Nummular chorioretinal depigmented scars, or
      2. RPE clumping, or
      3. Recurrent or chronic anterior uveitis
4. Neurological/auditory findings
   a. Meningismus
   b. Tinnitus
   c. Cerebrospinal fluid pleocytosis
5. Integumentary findings
   a. Alopecia
   b. Poliosis
   c. Vitiligo

Complete VKH requires 1 to 5. Incomplete VKH requires 1 to 3 and either 4 or 5. Probable VKH requires criteria 1 to 3 only.

7. Diagnostic Criteria

In 1980, the American Uveitis Society proposed a diagnostic criteria (Table 1) [5] taking into consideration those previously suggested by Sugiura (Table 2). However, this criteria come short in making diagnosis in the acute phase as 2 of the 4 criteria occur only be seen in the chronic phase (chronic bilateral iridociclytis and cutaneous signs). In an effort to unify concepts and allow the comparison of results from clinical studies from different countries, the International Committee on Nomenclature proposed the Revised Diagnostic Criteria for VKH disease in 2001 [4]. The Revised Diagnostic Criteria for VKH disease subdivides patients into 3 categories, namely probable, incomplete and complete. It encompasses a broader range of patients as the ocular manifestations may be either acute or chronic to met the criteria.

8. Differential Diagnosis

The principal differential diagnosis of VKH disease is sympathetic ophthalmia which prorogates the existence of previous ocular trauma or surgery. Other conditions that may mimic VKH disease are: acute posterior multifocal placoid pigmentar epitheliopathy (APMPPE), posterior scleritis, sarcoidosis, other white-dot syndromes, other conditions related to diffuse choroiditis and intraocular primary lymphoma (Table 4). Based on this, a complete history and physical examination followed by blood tests, tuberculin test, and image should be performed in all patients.

Table 4. Differential diagnosis of uveitis in the set of VKH disease

Sympathetic ophthalmia
Acute posterior multifocal placoid pigment epitheliopathy
Posterior scleritis
Multiple evanescent white dot syndrome
Tuberculosis
Sarcoidosis
Intraocular B-cell lymphoma
Metastatic carcinoma
Idiopathic uveal effusion syndrome

9. Prognosis

Systemic steroid treatment gives to two-thirds of the patients a fair visual prognosis, retaining 20 / 40 or better final visual acuity [16]. Fortunately, only the minority (11%) of these patients will have a visual acuity of 20 / 200 or worse.

10. Treatment and Complications

The standard therapy includes high dose of systemic corticosteroid besides topical medication for anterior uveitis. Prednisone should be used in a typical dosage of 1 to 2 mg/kg/day orally. There is no evidence of superiority of intravenous to oral use of corticosteroid. If the retinal detachment do not respond to oral corticosteroid therapy, intravenous methylprenisolone therapy is strongly suggested. Early steroid therapy followed by a slow taper in a period of 6 to 9 months is advised. This has shown to improve the prognosis by reducing the length of disease, the incidence of chronic phase and decreasing extra ocular manifestations in VKH disease.

In refractory cases or in those where it is necessary to withdraw the steroid administration more quickly it is important to use systemic immunosuppressants, such as cyclosporine, which is the most commonly used. However, the American Uveitis Society, and International Uveitis Study Group consensus panel after an evidence-based exercise reviewing literature, concluded that VKH may require immunosuppressant to control the inflammation [17, 18]. Other cytostatic agents may be used, such as cyclophosphamide, chlorambucil, azathioprine, and more recently, mycophenolate mofetil.

In a review of 13 patients, the authors compared patients who had undergone prolonged steroid therapy with or without the delayed addition of immunosuppressive drugs versus those who received prompt immune-suppressant (within 6 months). They found that 7 of 8 patients in the first group improved visual acuity from presentation whereas 3 of 5 without prompt immunossupressant suffered deterioration in final visual acuity [17].

Regarding biological therapy, a pilot study demonstrated that daclizumab (anti–interleukin-2 receptor antibody) seems to be safe and effective at controlling inflammation in a group of 10 uveitis patients that included 2 patients with VKH [19].

Choroidal neovascular membranes may be treated with traditional photocoagulation therapy or, more recently, with intraocular anti-angiogenic drug therapy. Acute angle closure glaucoma in the acute phase of the disease typically resolves after appropriate steroid treatment.

Cataract extraction in patients with uveitis can be challenging due to posterior synechiae and shallow anterior chamber. Synechiolysis, pupil stretching, and iris hooks may be necessary. Peripheral iridectomy should be considered in patients at risk for angle closure. The safety of intraocular lens use is not completely known. The authors stressed the importance of preoperative and postoperative control of inflammation, then it is recommended a period of at least 3-6 months of no acute ocular inflammation followed by one week of preoperative corticosteroids, with a postoperative tapering [7].

References

[1] Koyanagi YD. Alopecia und poliosis bei schwerer Uveitis nicht traumatischen Ursprungs. *Klin Monatsbl Augenkeikd* 1929;194:194-211.

[2] Vogt A. Fruhzeitiges Ergaruen der Zilien und Bemerkungen uber den sogenaten plotzlichen Eintreitt dieser Veranderung. *Klin Monatsbl Augenkeikd* 1906;44:228-42.

[3] Harada E. Acute diffuse choroiditis. *Acta Soc Ophtalmol Jpn* 1926;30:356-78.

[4] Read RW, Holland GN, Rao NA, et al. Revised diagnostic criteria for Vogt-Koyanagi-Harada disease: report of an international committee on nomenclature. *Am J Ophtalmol* 2001;131:647-52.

[5] Snyder DA, Tessler HH. Vogt-Koyanagi-Harada syndrome. *Am J ophthalmol* 1980;90:69-75.

[6] Belfort Junior R, Nishi M, Hayashi S, et al. Vogt-Koyanagi-Harada´s disease in Brazil. *Jpn J Ophthalmol* 1988;32:344-7.

[7] Moorthy RS Inomata J, Rao NA. (1995) Vogt-Koyanagi-Harada syndrome. *Surv Ophthalmol* 39:265–292.

[8] Damico FM, Cunha-Neto E, Goldberg AC, et al. T-cell recognition and cytokine profile induced by melanocyte epitopes inpatients with HLA-

DRB1*0405-positive and -negative Vogt-Koyanagi-Harada uveitis. *Invest Ophthalmol Vis Sci.* 2005;46:2465-71.

[9] Yamaki K, Gocho K, Hayakawa K, et al. Tyrosinase family proteins are antigens specific to Vogt-Koyanagi-Harada disease. *J Immunol* 2000;165:7323-9.

[10] Shindo Y, Ohno S, Yamamoto T, Nakamura S, Inoko H. Complete association of the HLA-DRB1*04 and –DQB1*04 alleles with Vogt-Koyanagi-Harada′s disease. *Hum Immunol* 1994;39:169-76.

[11] Goldberg AC, Yamamoto JH, Chiarella JM, et al. HLA-DRB1*0405 is the predominant allele in Brazilian patients with Vogt-Koyanagi-Harada disease. *Hum Immunol* 1998 ;59:183-8.

[12] de Smet MD, Yamamoto JH, Mochizuki M, Gery I, Singh VK, Shinohara T, Wiggert B, Chader GJ, Nussenblatt RB. Cellular immune responses of patients with uveitis to retinal antigens and their fragments. *Am J Ophthalmol* 199015;110(2):135-42.

[13] Chee S-P, Chi DL, Cheng CL, et al. Visual function in Vogt-Konayagi-Harada patients. *Graefe's Arch Clin Exp Ophthalmol* 2005;243; 785-790.

[14] da Silva FT, Damico FM, Marin ML, Goldberg AC, Hirata CE, Takiuti PH,Olivalves E, Yamamoto JH. Revised diagnostic criteria for Vogt Koyanagi-Harada disease: considerations on the different disease categories. *Am J Ophthalmol* 2009;147(2):339-345.

[15] M Shinzato, JH Yamamoto, CE Hirata, et al, Anti-SS-A/Ro reactivity in patients with Vogt-Koyanagi-Harada syndrome- *Lupus* 2004;13, 279-80.

[16] Yamamoto JH, Damico FM, Hirata CE, Kubo PY, Goldberg AC, Kalil J, Olivalves E. Epidemiological and clinical features of Brazilian patients with VKH syndrome. In: P*roceedings of the Vth International Symposium on Uveitis.* Dodds EM, Couto CA (eds). Elsevier Sci, BV, Amsterdam, p. 175, 2000.

[17] Paredes I, Ahmed M, Foster CS. Immunomodulatory therapy for VKH patients as first line therapy. *Ocul Immunol Inflamm.* 2006;14:87–90.

[18] Jabs DA, Rosenbaum JT, Foster CS, et al. Guidelines for the use of immunosuppressive drugs in patients with ocular inflammatory disorders: recommendations of an expert panel. *Am J Ophthalmol.* 2000;130:492–513.

[19] Nussenblatt RB, Fortin E, Schiffman R, et al. Treatment of noninfectious intermediate and posterior uveitis with the humanized

anti-Tac mAb: a phase I/II clinical trial. *Proc Natl Acad Sci USA*. 1999;96:7462–7466.

In: Advances in Eye Research. Volume 1 ISBN 978-1-61324-169-1
Editor: W. L. Thomsen, pp. 159-168

Chapter VIII

Uveitis in Rheumatology Practice: Current Concepts and Treatment

Alexandre Wagner Silva de Souza[1,*], *Jozelio de Carvalho*[2†], *Joyce Hisae Yamamoto*[3] *and Simone Appenzeller*[4,†]

[1]Assistant physician at Universidade Federal de São Paulo, Brasil
[2]Rheumatology Division University of São Paulo, School of Medicine, Brasil
[3]Department of Ophthalmology, University of São Paulo School of Medicine, Brasil
[4]Rheumatology Division, Faculty Medical Science, State University of Campinas, Brazil

* Corresponding author: Alexandre W. S. de Souza MD, PhD. Disciplina de Reumatologia, Universidade Federal de São Paulo, Rua Botucatu, 740, 3 andar, São Paulo – SP, Brasil, 04023-900. Telephone: 55-11-55764239; E-mail: alexandre_wagner@uol.com.br
† Carvalho J. F received grants from Federico Foundation and CNPq (300665/2009-1); Apenzeller S received grants from CNPq (2009/06049-6) and FAPESP (2008/02917-0).

Abstract

The eye is an essential organ for survival and is highly vulnerable to the destructive potential of immunogenic inflammation. Immune privilege of the eye has coped with the countermanding threats to vision of ocular infections and ocular immunity and inflammation. Among the primary features that account for its existence is the anterior chamber-associated immune deviation with a prolonged acceptance of solid tissue and tumor allografts in the anterior chamber and the induction of systemic tolerance to eye-derived antigens. Therefore, immune-mediated inflammation in the eye does not develop at the same pace as in other sites of the body. Uveitis is the most common autoimmune manifestation that affects the eye and may be an important cause of blindness among young individuals. The autoimmune nature of several uveitis is supported by experimental data from animal models, the presence of *in vitro* T lymphocytes responses to one or more retinal auto-antigens, the association of specific HLA molecules and the responsiveness to immunosuppressive drugs. Acute anterior uveitis is the main ocular manifestation of spondyloarthropathies in which uveitis can be the first manifestation of the disease. Precise patterns of uveitis are frequently associated with systemic diseases. Thus, the close collaboration between ophthalmologists and rheumatologists avoids unnecessary diagnostic tests and is essential for the correct assessment and treatment of these patients. Acute anterior uveitis usually has a good prognosis compared with other forms of uveitis. However, it is a cause of disability when flares are frequent. Small prospective studies conducted with sulphasalazine have demonstrated a reduction in the number of flares. Other patterns of uveitis have a worse prognosis, and systemic corticosteroids and/or immunosuppressive drugs are usually required.

The aim of this paper is to review the main rheumatological conditions associated with uveitis and discuss possible treatment strategies for these conditions.

Keywords: Uveitis, rheumatic diseases, systemic vasculitides

Introduction

Uveitis refers to inflammation of the pigmented vascular middle layer of the eye named uveal tract. The anterior portion of the uvea includes the iris and the ciliary body whereas its posterior portion is known as the choroid.

Uveitis may be classified based on the anatomical involvement of the eye into anterior, intermediate, posterior and panuveitis. There are several inflammatory and infectious causes of uveitis, in addition to ocular uveitic syndromes. It is the most common form of ocular inflammation and remains a significant cause of visual loss [1].

Uveitis is described in several rheumatologic disorders including spondyloarthritis, systemic autoimmune diseases and systemic vasculitides as well as in systemic chronic granulomatous diseases such as sarcoidosis [1,2]. Herein, we revise clinical manifestations and therapy of uveitis occurring in patients with rheumatic disorders.

Uveitis in Spondyloarthritis

Spondyloarthritis (SpA) is a heterogeneous group of diseases that include ankylosing spondylitis (AS), reactive arthritis (ReA), psoriatic arthritis, arthritis associated with inflammatory bowel disease and undifferentiated SpA. SpA share certain common clinical features such as inflammation of axial joints (especially the sacroiliac joints), asymmetric oligoarthritis mainly affecting the lower limbs, and enthesitis. Extra-articular manifestations of SpA include genital, skin and vascular lesions, eye and bowel inflammation. There is an association with preceding or ongoing infectious processes and strong association of SpA with the human leukocyte antigen (HLA) B27 [3].

Acute anterior uveitis is the most common extra-articular feature of SpA. In a recent systematic literature review, the mean prevalence of uveitis was 32.7% in SpA and it varied in different types of SpA. It was 36.9% in arthritis associated with inflammatory bowel disease, 33.2% in ankylosing spondylitis, 25.6% in reactive arthritis, 25.1% in psoriatic arthritis and 13.2% in undifferentiated SpA. The prevalence of uveitis increases with disease duration and HLA-B27 was associated with anterior uveitis with an odds ratio of 4.2 (95% confidence interval 3.3 to 5.3) [4,5].

The uveitis in SpA is acute in 88.7% and anterior in 90.5%. It is typically manifested by the sudden onset of unilateral pain and eye redness. Complete resolution is observed within several weeks. Recurrences often involve the contralateral eye and are observed in 50.6%. Reduction of visual activity occurs in only 8.3%. Posterior uveitis rarely occurs in patients with SpA [4,5].

Currently, the most employed therapy for acute anterior uveitis associated with SpA is topical corticosteroid with usually a good clinical response. Dilating eye drops are used to prevent synechiae and to relieve pain from ciliary muscle spasms. For persistent ocular inflammation despite topical therapy periocular injection or oral corticosteroids may be administered. Analysis of trials in AS patients have revealed a significant reduction in the rate of incidence of flares of uveitis with infliximab and adalimumab but not with etanercept [6].

Uveitis in Behçet's Disease

Behçet's disease (BD) is an inflammatory disorder characterized by recurrent oral aphthous ulcers, genital ulcers, ocular inflammation and skin lesions. Involvement of the gastrointestinal tract, central nervous system and large vessels in BD although occur less frequently, they are associated with higher morbidity [7,8].

In patients with BD the eye is involved in 30-70% of cases and it is commonly bilateral. The typical ocular manifestation is a chronic and relapsing non-granulomatous uveitis that may involve the anterior or posterior segment of the eye or both (panuveitis). Isolated anterior uveitis and/or hypopyon are observed in only a small fraction of patients. Other ocular manifestations of BD include retinal vasculitis, vitreous hemorrhage, vitritis, optic neuritis, retinal neovascularization and retinal vein occlusion [7-10].

Young males usually present a more severe eye involvement among BD patients. It generally occurs within three years after disease onset but may be the presenting feature of BD in 10-20% of patients. Recurrent attacks of ocular inflammation usually leads to significant morbidity and blindness may be observed in up to 25% of patients despite treatment [7-10].

Therapy of ocular manifestations of BD depends on the severity of eye involvement. The objective of the therapy for ocular manifestations of BD is to suppress inflammation and to prevent recurrent attacks, since they are associated with an increased risk of permanent blindness. Local and systemic corticosteroids are usually prescribed and rapidly suppress eye inflammation in BD especially in patients with the involvement of the anterior segment of the eye. However, whenever the posterior segment is affected the patient should be treated with systemic corticosteroids and azathioprine. The latter is widely accepted as the initial immunosuppressive agent for ocular involvement in BD based on the results of a randomized placebo controlled trial that showed that azathioprine (2.5mg/kg/day) decreased hypopyon uveitis attacks, stabilized visual acuity and decreased the development of new eye disease. The benefits of azathioprine continue on the long term [11].

If the patient presents severe eye disease or retinal involvement, it is recommended to use cyclosporine A (2-5mg/kg/day) or infliximab in combination with corticosteroids and azathioprine. Interferon (INF)α may be used in association with corticosteroids as an alternative [11].

Uveitis in Connective Tissue Diseases

Although uveitis is not a prominent feature of connective tissue diseases, some disorders develop important ocular manifestations even with sight-threatening complications. Sjögren`s syndrome is an important cause of keratoconjunctivitis sicca in either its primary form or in forms associated with rheumatoid arthritis (RA) and systemic lupus erythematosus (SLE). Scleritis is a severe of manifestation of RA and is usually seen in patients with advanced disease with other extra-articular features. It is secondary to vasculitis affecting the vascular plexuses of the sclera and episclera [2].

Systemic Lupus Erythematosus

SLE is a multisystem autoimmune disease with a broad range of clinical presentations. SLE is a chronic illness with periods of active disease and remission. It affects mainly young women during their reproductive ages when the women:men ratio reaches 9:1. The combination of suggestive clinical manifestations of SLE (e.g. nephritis, skin rashes, serositis and cytopenias) with the detection of autoantibodies such as antinuclear antibodies, anti-double strand DNA (dsDNA) and anti-Sm antibodies settles the correct diagnosis. SLE can be life-threatening when major organs are affected [12].

SLE may affect any part of the eye and the visual pathway; some manifestations are sight-threatening and reflect active systemic disease. Additionally, therapy used for SLE manifestations may cause ocular problems such as cataracts and retinopathy. Although choroidal disease is rare in SLE, retinal vascultis is a common ocular manifestation and occurs in up to 10% of patients. It is an arteriolar vasculitis that produces cotton wool spots and arterial occlusions. Retinal venulitis might also develop and both could result in substantial vision loss. It should be distinguished from hypertensive retinopathy, specially in patients with renal involvement, and from significant vaso-occlusive disease in the setting of the antiphospholipid syndrome. Other important ocular manifestations of SLE include secondary Sjögren's syndrome with keratoconjunctivitis sicca, scleritis, episcleritis and optic nerve disease [13].

Treatment of SLE depends on the severity of the disease. Corticosteroids as well as immunosuppressive agents such as cyclophosphamide, azathioprine and cyclosporine may be used in patients with SLE and sight-threatening disease [12,13].

Uveitis in Systemic Vasculitis

Primary systemic vasculitides are a heterogeneous group of diseases characterized by leukocyte infiltration of vessel walls leading either to destruction of vascular structures bleeding or to vascular occlusion resulting in downstream tissue ischemia and necrosis. The affected vessel may vary in size, type and localization. Multiple organs might be affected in different combinations. Although several classification systems have been developed, systemic vasculitides are usually classified according to the predominant size of vessels involved. Takayasu arteritis and giant cell arteritis are classified as large vessel vasculitis whereas polyarteritis nodosa, Kawasaki disease and primary central nervous system vasculitis are classified as medium-vessel vasculitis. Small vessel vasculitis include the so-called ANCA-associated vasculitis (e.g. Wegener's granulomatosis, microscopic polyangiitis and Churg-Strauss syndrome), cryoglobulinemic vasculitis, Henoch-Schönlein purpura and cutaneous leukocytoclastic vasculitis [14]. Uveitis and retinal vasculitis are not common features of systemic vasculitis, but may be observed in patients with Wegener's granulomatosis (WG), microscopic polyangiitis (MPA), Churg-Strauss syndrome (CSS) and polyarteritis nodosa (PAN) [2,15,16].

ANCA-Associated Vasculitis

Ophthalmic manifestations occur in up to 58% of patients with WG with 8% suffering disease-related vision loss. The most common manifestation in WG is orbital disease (15-20%) manifested as proptosis, painful extra-ocular muscle weakness or orbital mass. Scleral involvement is another prevalent ocular manifestation in WG with episcleritis occurring in 3.5% and scleritis in up to 15% of cases. Both necrotizing and non-necrotizing scleritis can be seen, often associated with peripheral keratitis. Eyelids may also be involved in patients with WG and it is usually manifested as dacryoadenitis, dacrocystitis, nasolacrimal obstruction, eyelid ulceration and fistula formation. Uveitis is not a common feature of WG (2.9%). Anterior, posterior or panuveitis may occur. However, retinal or choroidal vasculitis is the most common intraocular feature of WG. It is important to reassure that signs of ocular inflammation in WG may be the clue for disease activity in other organs and it should trigger prompt investigation to determine the extent of the disease [15,16].

Ocular disease is less common in patients with MPA. In a cohort study of 85 patients with MPA, confirmed in most cases by biopsy, only one had ocular disease. Scleritis and retinal vasculitis are the most frequent ocular manifestations of MPA, but episcleritis, conjunctivitis and peripheral ulcerative keratitis have been described [16,17].

Induction therapy for systemic GW and MPA includes high dose corticosteroids and cyclophosphamide for 3-6 months, followed by azathioprine or methotrexate to maintain remission. Patients with localized WG may be treated with corticosteroids and methotrexate [18]. Recently, rituximab has been shown to be not inferior to cyclophosphamide in patients with systemic WG and MPA in placebo controlled randomized trials [19,20].

Patients with CSS may also present ocular manifestations, especially retinal vasculitis with retinal vein and/or artery occlusion. Orbital disease is also an important ocular feature of CSS, it is manifested by dacryoadenitis or myositis. Orbital disease in CSS is associated with a good prognosis and all patients reported in literature have maintained a good visual acuity [16]. Treatment of CSS is guided by the presence of prognostic factors, the so-called five-factor score (FFS) that include serum creatinine level > 1.58mg/dL, proteinúria >1g per day, gastrointestinal tract involvement, cardiomyopathy and central nervous system involvement. Patients without prognostic factors have a 5-year mortality rate of 11.9% are treated only with high-dose corticosteroids. Patients with at least one prognostic factor have a 5-year mortality rate of 25.9-46% and are treated with high-dose corticosteroids and cyclophosphamide [21].

Polyarteritis Nodosa

Ocular involvement in PAN is uncommon and consists of retinal vasculitis, scleritis, peripheral ulcerative keratitis or orbital inflammation presented as proptosis. Similarly to CSS, treatment of PAN is based on the presence of prognostic factors on FFS [2,22].

Kawasaki Disease

In patients with Kawasaki disease conjunctival injection occurs due to vasculitis of conjunctival vessels. A small number of patients may also develop anterior uveitis. Both uveitis and conjunctivitis usually resolve with topical corticosteroids. Intravenous immunoglobulin combined with high-dose aspirin are used for systemic manifestations and reduces the incidence of coronary artery aneurysms [2,23].

References

[1] Srivastava A, Rajappa M, Kaur J. Uveitis: mechanisms and recent advances in therapy. *Clin Chim Acta* 2010;411(17-18):1165-71.

[2] McCluskey P, Powell RJ. The eye in systemic inflammatory diseases. *Lancet* 2004;364:2125-33.

[3] Sieper J, Rudwaleit M, Khan MA, Braun J. Concepts and epidemiology of spondyloarthritis. *Best Pract Res Clin Rheumatol* 2006;20:401-17.

[4] Zeboulon N, Dougados M, Gossec L. Prevalence and characteristics of uveitis in the spondyloarthropathies: a systematic literature review. *Ann Rheum Dis* 2008;67:955-9.

[5] Martin TM, Smith JR, Rosenbaum JT. Anterior uveitis: current concepts of pathogenesis and interactions with the spondylo-arthropathies. *Curr Opin Rheumatol* 2002;14:337-41.

[6] Elewaut D, Matucci-Cerinic M. Treatment of ankylosing spondylitis and extra-articular manifestations in everyday rheumatology practice. *Rheumatology (Oxford)* 2009;48:1029-35.
[7] Mendes D, Correia M, Barbedo M, et al. Behçet`s disease – A contemporary review. *J Autoimmun* 2009;32:178-88.
[8] Yurdakul S, Yazici H. Behçet`s syndrome. *Best Pract Res Clin Rheumatol* 2008;22:793-809.
[9] Tugal-Tutkun I, Onal S, Altan-Yaycioglu R, Huseyin Altunbas H, Urgancioglu M. Uveitis in Behçet disease: an analysis of 880 patients. *Am J Ophthalmol* 2004;138:373-80.
[10] Nobuyoshi K, Miyazaki A, Iwata D, Ohno S, Stansford MR, Chams H. Ocular features of Behçet`s disease: an international collaborative study. *Br J Ophthalmol* 2007;91:1579-82.
[11] Hatemi G, Silman A, Bang D, et al. Eular recommendations for the management of Behçet disease. *Ann Rheum Dis* 2008;67:1656-62.
[12] D`Cruz DP, Khamashta MA, Hughes GR. Systemic lupus erythematosus. *Lancet* 2007;369:587:96.
[13] Sivaraj RR, Durrani OM, Denniston AK, Murray PI, Gordon C. Ocular manifestations of systemic lupus erythematosus. *Rheumatology (Oxford)* 2007;46:1757-62.
[14] Watts RA, Scott DG. Recent developments in the classification and assessment of vasculitis. *Best Pract Res Clin Rheumatol* 2009;23:429-43.
[15] Tarabishy AB, Schulte M, Papaliodis GN, Hoffman GS. Wegener`s granulomatosis: clinical manifestations, differential diagnosis, and management of ocular and systemic disease. *Surv Ophthalmol* 2010;55:429-444.
[16] Kubal AA, Perez VL. Ocular manifestations of ANCA-associated vasculitis. *Rheum Dis Clin N Am* 2010;36:573-86.
[17] Guillevin L, Durand-Gasselin B, Cevallos R, et al. Microscopic polyangiitis: clinical and laboratory findings in eighty-five patients. *Arthritis Rheum* 1999;42(3): 421–3.
[18] Mukhtyar C, Guillevin L, Cid MC, et al. Eular recommendations for the management of primary small and medium vessel vasculitis. *Ann Rheum Dis* 2009;68:310-7.
[19] Stone JH, Merkel PA, Spiera R, et al. Rituximab versus cyclophosphamide for ANCA-associated vasculitis. *N Eng J Med* 2010;363:221-32.

[20] Jones RB, Tervaert JWC, Hauser T, et al. Rituximab versus cyclophophamide in ANCA-associated renal vasculitis. *N Eng J Med* 2010;363:211-20.
[21] Sinico RA, Bottero P. Churg-Strauss angiitis. *Best Pract Res Clin Rheumatol* 2009;23:355-66.
[22] Guillevin L, Lhote F, Gayraud M, et al. Prognostic factors in polyarteritis nodosa and Churg-Strauss syndrome. A prospective study in 342 patients. *Medicine (Baltimore)* 1996;75:17-28.
[23] Williams RV, Minich LL, Tani LY. Pharmacological therapy for patients with Kawasaki disease. *Pediatr Drugs* 2001;3:649-60.

Index

F

G

J

K

L

N

O

P

R

S

T

U

V

W

Y